MW00438383

Recognizing Reality

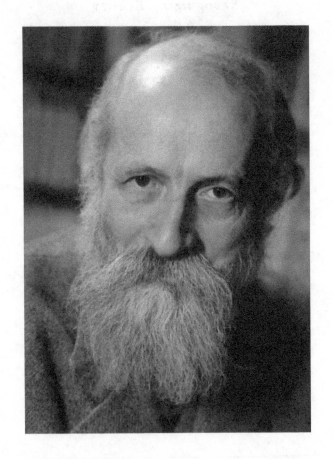

Martin Buber (1878, Vienna–1965, Jerusalem)

Recognizing Reality

Youth Education
in a Time of Global Crisis

Peter Selg

SteinerBooks | 2022

STEINERBOOKS
AN IMPRINT OF ANTHROPOSOPHIC PRESS, INC.
P.O. BOX 58, Hudson, NY 12534
www.steinerbooks.org

Copyright © 2022 by Peter Selg. All rights reserved. No
part of this publication may be reproduced, stored in a
retrieval system, or transmitted, in any form or by any
means, electronic, mechanical, photocopying, recording, or otherwise, without the prior written permission of
the publisher. This book was originally published as two
volumes in German as *Wirklichkeits-verständnis: Jugend-
pädagogik in globaler Krisenzeit* and as *Zivilcourage: Die
Herausforderung Freier Waldorfschulen* (Verlag des Ita
Wegman Instituts, Arlesheim, Switzerland, 2021).

Translated by Jeff Martin

Design by William Jens Jensen

LIBRARY OF CONGRESS CONTROL NUMBER: 2022939272

ISBN: 978-1-62148-308-3

Printed in the United States of America

Contents

Foreword

The following text is the written version of a presentation I had planned to give last December (2020) at a symposium on the developmental and educational problems and challenges of the Covid crisis. However, due to the second "lockdown," the event had to be cancelled on short notice and has not been rescheduled since. On the appointed day of the symposium, however, I wrote down—for what it was worth—approximately what I had wanted to say.

Originally, I wanted to refrain from publishing it. The pressure on Waldorf schools and teaching staffs is already extraordinarily great—between parents who (until the school was closed again) demanded even more and stricter hygiene measures and, if necessary, reported their own child's school to the authorities, and parents for whom the existing school rules went much too far and exceeded the pedagogical requirements. And all this under the scrutiny of a local and national press that once again takes aim at Waldorf schools and puts some of their critical teachers and parents in the category of contrarians, "Covid deniers," and "covidiots," or among right-wing *Reichsbürger* [citizens of the

Reich]* extremists, and once again puts the whole of Anthroposophy under general suspicion. Furthermore, it was, and is, clear to me that my thoughts and considerations by no means represent "the" point of view of Waldorf education, that I am not an upper school teacher, and that I do not work in the reality of a school under the conditions of the current crisis.

However, the other speakers of the cancelled symposium, to whom I sent the text, were *in favor* of its publication after reading it. Also, some other friends who learned of it in the meantime were of the opinion that shutting up and keeping silent cannot be the solution in a widely muddled situation, but only clear thoughts and dialogues can enable and shape the future. However, these undoubtedly presuppose a critical analysis of the present situation and its problems.

Thus, I have finally decided to publish the text, as a continuation of what has already been elaborated at a Stuttgart pedagogical colloquium in July 2020,[1] together with various other approaches and essays for understanding our present situation.[2]

I am also sure that in the near future, critical evaluations of the overall sequence of events since February 2020 will be formulated, and differentiated perspectives will be of interest. The anthroposophic movement has

---

*   *Reichsbürger* is a term used in Germany for groups and individuals who reject the legitimacy of the modern German state, the Federal Republic of Germany, and maintain that the German Reich (1871–1945) continues to exist, governed by a *Kommissarische Reichsregierung* (*KRR*, Provisional Reich Government) or *Exilregierung* ("government-in-exile").

something essential to contribute[3] and little or nothing to do with how it is being characterized in the media.

Anthroposophy has nothing to do with the "AfD" and the *"Reichsbürger,"* with right-wing nationalist and right-wing extremist, racist and anti-Semitic circles and forces—these have been among its fiercest enemies from the beginning.[4] It represents a genuine science of freedom, relies on wide-awake forces of individuality and the dignity of every human being, and helps to prepare a socially and ecologically oriented civil society of the future.

Peter Selg
Casa Andrea Cristoforo
Ascona, January 31, 2021

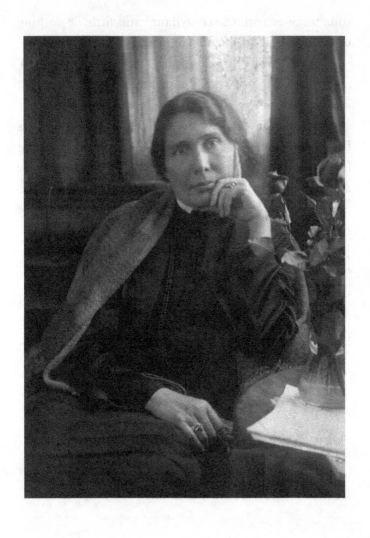

Ita Wegman, 1928
© *Ita Wegman Archiv, Arlesheim*

On the "Right to Education"

On November 24, 2020, *Der Spiegel* (online) published an article with the headline "Wie Schüler alleingelassen werden" [How students are left alone] about a senior at a Waldorf school in southern Germany who called the police to the school because he had encountered a teacher without a mask and confronted her (she had a medical certificate). The author of the lurid newspaper report, Swantje Unterberg, concluded, "Students are largely on their own [at the Waldorf school] when they stand up for the mask requirement and thus for their right to education." She also reported on an open letter from the student council at the same Waldorf school, in which students had urged all teachers "to maintain the minimum distance required by law or to pursue homeschooling."

I wondered, as I read the article, about the state of mind, the mood of life, and the worldview of the youth who called in the police to crack down on a teacher without a mask. Where are the young people today? What happened, and how could such an escalated situation develop in a relatively short time—a situation that would have been completely unthinkable a year ago? Why does a Waldorf student call the police at the sight of a maskless teacher? Even though the student obviously appeared to be quite self-confident, I suspect that—in addition to the youthful gesture of rebellion—considerable insecurity and fear played a role, which would not be surprising after the media coverage of the last eight months. I assume that it was also about the search for stability, security, and clarity in a complicated situation. The distance requirement and the mask requirement now seem reasonable to young people; they satisfy the age-appropriate need for rationality, the comprehensible logic of combating or containing the virus, which has been so often outlined in the media.

The logic of "equal rights for all" will also have played a role in this instance—the need for equal treatment or at least for comprehensible transparency of the situation. Young people have submitted to the mask requirement, the rationality of which seems plausible to them; but they have also accepted it because of the appeal to protect others, especially the old and the weak, which has not passed them by without leaving a trace. Perhaps also because they want to make at least their modest contribution and signal that they are prepared to sacrifice—and because of the extreme social pressure to conform. In the media, people without masks have been and continue to be presented to them almost exclusively as "Covid deniers," "covidiots," social egoists, enemies of science, right-wing extremists, unworldly mystics ("esotericists"), or potential murderers—usually all of these at the same time—essentially, as crazy or deliberately reckless endangerers of the common good who possibly belong in psychiatric care or in prison. Against this background, the teenager's reaction seems understandable.

However, perhaps he would have been able to understand or accept or at least tolerate the teacher's position, her view of the overall situation, and her inner attitude, if it had been presented to him personally, explained calmly and authentically—or if the teacher's attitude and position had occupied a different space in the general consciousness, thus also in the media landscape, if it had different and equally weighted media coverage. In my experience, young people have the ability to change perspectives and also to tolerantly accept other views and attitudes to life, as long as these are made sufficiently clear to them, whether from the other person's own perspective or from general education.

They are by no means intolerant, as long as they can see the different positions in their uniqueness and inner validity. However, deeper conversations of this kind, personal discussions about the Covid situation and each person's perception or experience of it—as well as differentiated media reports that include multiple perspectives—have been almost absent or have become impossible since spring 2020. Waldorf schools are no exception but are a mirror of society. There, too, silence has fallen over the biggest and most important, all-determining, and changing topic. That which shapes the lives of everyone—the Covid crisis—cannot be discussed because the social mood is so emotional and so radicalized, because the tension is too great. The most important questions become taboo. And in the end, the police come.

The "right" of young people "to education" was referred to in the above-mentioned report by the *Spiegel* journalist. I ask myself whether this "education" does not first and foremost include the present situation—at least in all upper schools, state and private, and thus also in Waldorf schools. According to Rudolf Steiner, the education of young people in Waldorf schools should be oriented toward "placing people into this world." If this does not succeed, "Waldorf School" will remain a mere "phrase."[5] "Into this world"—but this also means into this historical situation, which must be understood, within which one must orient oneself, the mastering of which is demanded of us, of all of us. Steiner goes on to say that Waldorf education in adolescence is about "awakening" education; about gaining a "broader horizon for life," not about "breaking away from the developments of the times." It is urgent for young people to understand the concrete "present," the "very, very nearness...of life."[6] Therefore, I think that there is not only a "right to education," to a "comprehensive" education, but even the obligation to it, if one does not want to break away from the "developments of the times," out of the "very, very nearness of life."

In contrast to the *Spiegel* author, however, I am of the well-founded opinion that the reporting of the so-called mainstream media, including the *Spiegel*, in the last eight months has not been conducive to providing a sufficient—and sufficiently differentiated—picture of the "developments of the times," a real insight into what is happening. This was different in the past, with *Der Spiegel, Der Zeit, Süddeutsche Zeitung,* and *Die Tageszeitung.* Schools are "educational institutions"— and as I already asserted in July 2020 at a colloquium in Stuttgart, in my opinion it is one of the tasks of Waldorf schools—especially in view of the one-sided, polarizing, and generally superficial and sensational reporting of the mainstream media—to contribute something essential to contemporary education. I said at that time that Waldorf schools should make an effort to raise the social level of the Covid discussion, at least in their own field, and to bring out the differentiated nature of the difficult situation—for example, through the quality of their approach to contemporary studies for high school students in various subjects, but perhaps also through events for parents and interested parties, inviting knowledgeable speakers from various areas of life and with different perspectives.[7]

I am convinced—perhaps naively or mistakenly— that through more knowledge, more comprehensive and complex knowledge, the rifts in society, and thus also in the school community, can be overcome through this step forward and toward the matter at hand, but by no means through a militant tabooing of the topic, through a tacit "Covid" ban on thought and speech. I am counting on this possibility of understanding—even if the assessments of the danger of the SARS-CoV-2 virus and the measures deemed necessary do not coincide at the moment. Amartya Kumar Sen, the Indian economist and philosopher, said on October 18, 2020, in St. Paul's Church in Frankfurt, when accepting the Peace Prize of the German Book Trade, that it is a matter of "reading" more, "talking" more, and "arguing" more.[8] Although his published speech is entitled "Die Pandemie des Autoritarismus" [The pandemic of authoritarianism], it has nothing superficially to do with *the* pandemic that is currently being talked about almost exclusively among us, the SARS-CoV-2 pandemic. Nevertheless, I would like to follow his advice in this difficult area as well: We need to read more, talk more, and argue more, by which Sen probably did not mean a spiteful fight, polemics, or hatred, but the airing of a genuine intellectual controversy.

I mentioned before the title of the report in *Spiegel* (online): "Wie Schüler alleingelassen werden" [How students are left alone]. I do indeed mean that they are mostly left very much alone with the subject of COVID-19, a subject about which, however, there is obviously nothing to discuss from the perspective of the *Der Spiegel* author, because everything is simple and crystal clear—her accusation of "being left alone" referred only to the observance or non-observance of the official hygiene regulations. However, I believe that students today need a new orientation to reality in order to reestablish their confidence in life and the world. They, and all of us, need to *know more*—and I would like to define and sketch out a few areas below that I believe should *also* be addressed. My list will be anything but complete. At the end of my remarks, I would like to briefly report on what I expect in pedagogical terms from this extended knowledge, which developmental abilities I have in mind, and what path into the future I see—especially, although by no means exclusively, for Waldorf schools and their young people. In a letter written in 1931—more than ninety years ago—to the Stuttgart Waldorf teacher Ernst Lehrs, Ita Wegman emphasized that "we must be careful that we do not gradually lose the youth, also the youth who have attended the Waldorf School, and also the youth who are still in the Waldorf School. Every soul is being fought for."[9]

Thus, in the following, I would like to outline some areas of knowledge and inherent problems that seem essential to me. Almost all of them seem to me to be of importance even beyond the acute crisis and to a large extent regardless of whether one considers the Covid policies to be right or wrong, to be the only way or changeable. I trust, as I said before, that this larger and wider, more complex knowledge will help us all and can create something unifying. By a "broader horizon for life," Steiner by no means meant only beautiful things. The "developments of the times" have their abysses, which must be known, also by young people, perhaps especially by young people. When I mention below some of the difficult areas and challenges that, in my opinion, young people should know about to gain a more differentiated assessment and evaluation of the situation—and also to overcome socially polar positions that lack mutual understanding—I do not mean, of course, that one should "lecture" them about these things. One can deal with these topics in class from different perspectives and with different questions, also with the help of different methods; one can bring interesting sources, texts, pictures, and video material, with which the students can actively work in small groups and in other forms. It is not about "teaching" but about working with the content. I will not go into pedagogical questions in the following and I am not a teacher; nevertheless, as I said, everything presented here seems important to me, otherwise I would not discuss it.

Knowing about the Disease

I'll start with the disease in question, which I believe young people in our schools should already be hearing more about, though not in a sensational way. It is important to understand that the COVID-19 disease is a medical reality and, like all humankind's diseases, has its own diverse manifestations, processes, and set of conditions—also with regard to the different ways in which people are affected. I do not mean that school-children should be confronted with all the details; they are not studying medicine and have already seen enough pictures from the ICU, and perhaps also heard interviews with those affected or their relatives. Nevertheless—or precisely because of this—I think it is important to talk to them about the phenomena and the variety of courses it takes: It is a viral respiratory infection, through a pathogen from the large group of coronaviruses, that takes its course harmlessly in most people, without any symptoms or with minor symptoms, and in other people severely or even very severely, mostly (although by no means without exception) in older people with pre-existing medical conditions or in people whose immune system is already very weakened, in which a variety of factors play a role.

COVID-19, as we all know, is a clinical reality, and those severely affected by it take an exceedingly hard road under intensive care treatments. Often all efforts end fatally. Nevertheless, the SARS-CoV-2 virus is not a demonic entity, and even the severe cases are by no means unique and completely beyond comparison. It is also good for young people to know how differently the disease runs its course in different countries and why that might be the case—there are, after all, a variety of experiences connected with something we call by the same name. In my opinion, young people should also know that, according to Georg Soldner, this disease represents an attack on the middle sphere of the human being *and* of society; we are all experiencing the latter at the moment, although the question is naturally what part is played by the disease and what part by the defenses erected against the pandemic. In this context, COVID-19 is not the only disease that can aggressively affect the human respiratory system.

In 2017 alone, according to WHO figures, eight hundred thousand children under the age of five died from lung infections worldwide. In Germany, influenza took the lives of more than twenty thousand people three years ago; and this was by no means the only severe flu epidemic in recent memory. One should not set these numbers against each other, but students should, I think, know something of the reality and prevalence of other diseases in the midst of the daily Covid numbers. "Tunnel vision," fixating solely on COVID-19, is unhelpful. We need more context, even in medical terms. But what newspaper currently reports on the approximately nine million people who die of cancer each year worldwide, a great many of whom could be saved by timely countermeasures and a change in social, socioeconomic, and socioecological conditions? Who is currently reporting how many lives could be saved by a significant reduction in particulate pollution? How many—or rather how few—headlines are made by multidrug-resistant hospital germs, which are connected with the abuse of antibiotics in factory farming and which, according to various reports, kill significantly more people per year than COVID-19 has so far?

It is important to understand the diseases, as well as infections and pollutants, with which we already live—and that by no means only COVID-19 but also the flu is regularly classified as a pandemic and also often causes long-lasting complaints and sometimes also organic consequential damages. Clemens G. Arvay has described this in his important, calm, and differentiated book, *Wir können es besser: Wie Umweltzerstörung die Corona-Pandemie auslöste und warum ökologische Medizin unsere Rettung ist* [We can do better: How environmental destruction triggered the Covid pandemic and why ecological medicine is our salvation], and it is well worth reading, even for young people.

None of this changes the grave reality of the COVID-19 disease, but it may well change something about our fixation on COVID, about our near-total banishment of other issues. As a trained specialist in child and adolescent psychiatry and psychotherapy, I would also like to say that children and adolescents should not be given the impression that something sinister has arisen out of nowhere, erupting into the hitherto perfect human world, simply because the infection and death rates of other diseases have not been published daily and carried to the last corner of the earth in sensational exhibitions.

Nor should they get the impression that a horrifying "killer virus" from China has suddenly come to us and to them via bats, a sinister micro-organism from the equally sinister genus of viruses, presented in a science-fiction-like manner, which is now threatening their grandparents—the greatest threat coming from the grandchildren themselves. Instead, children and young people should, in my opinion, also hear something from the field of biology about the positive significance of omnipresent viruses for human evolution, for our genome, and also for the maturation of our immune system. They should know—and really *sense and feel*—that viruses are not "evil" but a part of our organism, of our organic "self," and that also the group of mutable coronaviruses has been known for many years; we also live with them and deal with them, especially in the upper respiratory tract, although not with SARS-CoV-2, which is a new challenge for the human immune system, though not quite as new as initially assumed.

As I said, none of this changes the severity of many clinical cases of the disease we refer to as COVID-19, but it does change something about young people's attitude to life, their relationship to the world in which they live and in which they grow up, into which they grow. From the perspective of pedagogy and developmental psychology, it is this world that matters most. Is this world to be trusted, or is it essentially a place of insidious viruses that have infected humans via bats and have been traveling from person to person ever since, so that each person can bring death to the other, at any time and in any encounter? A place of demonic pathogens from which we can only protect ourselves, at least temporarily, through isolation or vaccination? And can this disease really be temporary at all? Is every other person a threat to me, especially without a mask? What kind of world do we live in?

Recognizing Connections

The Pandemic and the Environmental Scandal

A significant insight into one aspect of the world in which we live was provided in the summer of 2020 by medical ecologist Clemens G. Arvay in the book I mentioned. Among other things, he talks about the fact that a large number of the viral diseases caused by zoonoses—including very probably COVID-19—are the result of destructive human interventions in ecological contexts. There is a great deal of well-founded scientific literature beyond Arvay that corroborates this. We know that viral activity increases in biological systems that come under high stress; the previously existing equilibria changes between viruses and their hosts. Viruses can, of necessity, change their hosts; their release through the destruction of ecosystems and natural habitats has been demonstrated not only in connection with the genesis of HIV but also with the numerous cholera epidemics that ravaged Europe from the nineteenth century onward (including the one from which Hegel died in Berlin). The diseases of nature that humanity produces ultimately strike back at us in the form of the smallest and oldest life forms on the planet—viruses. Humanity produces these diseases through the industrial over-exploitation of rainforests and other natural habitats, through our lifestyle demands—including exorbitant meat consumption in wealthy, industrialized nations and the practice of factory farming—and through the manufacturing methods by which countless luxury products are made. Zoonoses arise when ecosystems are damaged and viruses are forced to jump to other host organisms—and it has been proven that ecologization and de-industrialization of agriculture and livestock are among the most effective protections against pandemics. The loss of biodiversity, the variety of species and their complex relationships, is momentous, and the consequences are increasingly dramatic. Pandemics are also among these consequences.

In my opinion, all of this must be talked about in high school classes; it belongs, I believe, to the "right to education," including "world education," and it belongs to the necessary awareness of the present, of the reality in which we and our fellow human beings live. It is important to know that the terrible Ebola epidemics in Central and West Africa are demonstrably related to the destruction of the rainforest, especially by U.S. and Chinese corporations, and that, most recently in 2018 in the Congo, with a seventy percent mortality rate, it was primarily children who died, largely because of internal bleeding. The aid organization Doctors without Borders called for an intensive aid effort by wealthy, industrialized nations, which as "externalization societies"—living at the expense of other societies and the natural environment—have significantly contributed to the suffering caused by the epidemic. This organization's call for help found only marginal resonance; the WHO was also part of this "global alliance of inaction." In this case, Europe, which was not affected by Ebola, did not point to the "value of every human life" that takes precedence over economics—something that has been repeated time and again since March 2020. One can argue that human communities usually only react when they themselves are endangered and affected; however, one should not be surprised if not everyone believes the moral appeals of governments and the institutional ethics of a global organization such as the WHO, and if doubts arise about the motives guiding their actions. Why double standards for those beyond the "external borders" of Europe and those within Europe itself? Such questions are of interest, and many sensitive young people asked them even before Covid, in the time of "Fridays for Future" and other humanitarian protests.

It should be noted at this point that the Covid crisis is also an "environmental scandal" (Arvay) and has to do with the severely injured biosphere of the living earth. A knowledge of the destructive system of the "externalization society" (Stephan Lessenich) belongs, in my opinion, to the necessary educational goals of an "age of extremes," in the "Anthropocene." "Thus, Covid is a direct consequence of our harmful abuse of nature" (Soldner).[10] Paul Schreyer speaks of the Covid crisis as a crisis of "ideology" rather than a new virus. Navid Kermani, in his speech in Bad Homburg a few weeks ago, quoted Hölderlin on the occasion of his 250th birthday: "The springs of the earth and the morning dew refresh your grove; can you do that, too? Alas! You can kill, but you can't create life."

I think it is also important to talk to young people about the history of science, which stands in the background of this domination of nature, about the teachings of Francis Bacon and René Descartes at the turn of the sixteenth and seventeenth centuries, about Descartes' powerful conception of the human being as the "master" and "owner" of nature, about the distinct attributes of this kind of knowledge for the sake of domination that emerged at that time and created the ideological and also methodological preconditions for technological materialism. As Charles Eisenstein wrote recently, in a simple and succinct manner:

> Just as it is a lot easier to degrade, to exploit, and to kill a person when one sees the victim as less than human, so too it is easier to kill Earth's beings when we see them as unliving and unconscious already. The clearcuts, the strip mines, the drained swamps, the oil spills, and so on are inevitable when we see Earth as a dead thing, insensate, an instrumental pile of resources.... If we see the world as dead, we will kill it.[11]

Moreover, I think it is important to speak in high school and in the context of Covid about the consequences of the ideology of unconditional economic growth, which turns nature into a "product," establishes an "it" relationship (in Martin Buber's terminology) to the natural environment, and sets in motion a dynamic of power and conquest that pushes democracy to its limits—where forces other and more powerful than parliaments and constitutions determine the playing field. Most young people are currently aware of the climate breakdown. But have they been given sufficient opportunity by teachers and parents, indeed by our educational institutions, to develop an overview of the causes and effects of the climate catastrophe, even though such an analysis of root causes seriously calls into question our current economic and social model and its philosophical underpinnings? Are young people sufficiently capable of linking problem areas, of seeing them in their context? Are we?

Already today, more than seventy million people are on the run because of climate changes and catastrophes; in 2050, floods are expected to make land areas uninhabitable where 350 million people currently live. It is now well known what share of the responsibility for this situation is borne by large corporations, especially through the over-exploitation of fossil fuels, and what role is played by the lifestyles of wealthy, industrialized nations—but also, what sums of money profit-driven corporations have invested over decades to suppress studies on climate change or to render them harmless through pseudo-scientific counter-arguments. These connections are known to experts in the field and it is not a "conspiracy theory." There is now consensus not only among climate researchers.

But where is the connection with the current pandemic, the young people will perhaps ask, but possibly also see it themselves: "one earth" also means "one health." "They [the children and young people] have been born into a future that can no longer be saved, but at most endured," said Navid Kermani in his Hölderlin speech, recounting the experience with his two daughters of watching David Attenborough's *A Life on Our Planet*, which, as a Netflix documentary, already had one million views after four hours.[12]

Countless young people are aware of the global crisis and the almost hopeless climate situation—perhaps that is why they follow the Covid rules so calmly, because they can do something simple here, can do something pragmatic, when the big picture seems so hopelessly muddled and can no longer be "saved." Perhaps, however, through a differentiated and engaging lesson—on the level of Attenborough—they could also be won over to insights into the interrelationships of ecological epidemiology, to an expanded knowledge of the relation of our interventions in ecosystems with the emergence of new diseases and also of the proven impairment of immune functions by environmental stresses, which played a not-insignificant role in the severe Covid cases in the Lombardy region of Italy and in other places, other "hotspots." At the end of a lecture on medical aspects of the Covid crisis, Georg Soldner said at the Goetheanum:

> We can promote health sustainably only if we take the health of animals, plants, and soil as seriously as our own. We need a science of the living; we need a maturation of our economy into an economy of common good. Believe me, the crucial answers to COVID-19 are not purely medical ones; they affect all areas of life and all of us who bear responsibility for this Earth and the generations that will follow us.[13]

Ecology, as a relational science, is of interest to many young people, as the recent Shell Youth Study shows. COVID-19, however, has something to do with the sickness of planet Earth, even if the mass media rarely illuminates this connection. To the extent that we, as educators and teachers, succeed in showing children and young people the corresponding connections, the simple—far too simple—polarizations (for or against the "Covid measures") recede into the background. There emerges instead a willingness to share responsibility for the future of civilization and life on Earth and to participate in changing the conditions that create the problems in the first place.

If, on the other hand, we simply accept masks, social distancing, and vaccination in order to return as quickly as possible to the so-called normality of a thoroughly pathological situation, we will have learned little or nothing from COVID-19, despite immeasurable damage. I think that this insight belongs to today's necessary "general education."

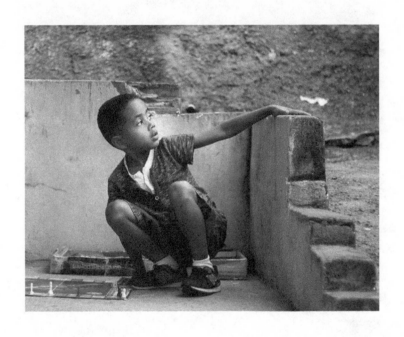

*A child in front of the music school of the favela Monte Azul,
São Paulo, Brazil, 2017 (Photo: Lina Selg)*

The Social Scandal

The socioeconomic reality of the world today shows how pathological our seeming "normality" is—and, in my opinion, young people in the third decade of the twenty-first century should also become aware of this aspect of reality, and consequently also of the COVID-19 reality. According to calculations by the organization Oxfam, already in 2015 sixty-two people—multibillionaires—owned as much wealth as half the world's population combined, or about 3.5 billion people.

In 2014, there were eighty billionaires who owned this much wealth, but by 2017, there were reportedly only eight. According to a study by the major bank UBS and the consulting firm PWC, which was published in October 2020 in Switzerland, the total wealth of the approximately 2,200 billionaires worldwide has increased rapidly during the COVID-19 pandemic—to a total of 10.2 trillion dollars.[14] As a reminder, a trillion is a million million. More telling, or at least somewhat more conceivable, was a report in *Die Tageszeitung* on December 10, 2020, quoting US research by the Institute for Policy Studies and a US tax justice organization, according to which the wealth of the approximately 650 billionaires in the US increased by one trillion dollars during the COVID-19 pandemic to a total of approximately four trillion dollars—that is, by no less than a quarter! Neither publication speculated about the backgrounds of this enormous growth during the pandemic but merely presented this fact of the immense, unimaginable profit of the most powerful—in particular, many large corporations in the tech industry, digital enterprises, and the operators of large online platforms, as well as the pharmaceutical industry.

The overall socioeconomic situation of the world's population is not only scandalous but highly pathogenic, disease-causing, and disease-sustaining; the COVID-19 disease in its worst forms also finds its suitable breeding ground in this extraordinary inequality of resources. A handful of powerful people own trillions while a billion others eke out a meager existence. According to WHO figures, 822 million people suffer from hunger worldwide. Nine million die of starvation every year without any "live update" reports and without a permanent media presence, without triple-digit billions in aid and international crisis teams. Among these figures are five to six million children. At the same time, there is agreement within the WHO and among other experts that there is enough food for the entire world population. It is a problem of the just distribution of resources, of nutrition, of the destruction of immense amounts of food in wealthy industrialized nations, of the industrial and increasingly climatic destruction of agricultural land in developing countries, etc. According to UNICEF, approximately fifteen thousand children under the age of five die of starvation or preventable diseases every day; their fate does not appear in the mass media, while the first children and adolescents with COVID-19 symptoms were sought out internationally by major media outlets.

Jean Ziegler, who was UN correspondent on the right to food from 2000 to 2008, estimates that approximately fifty million people die each year worldwide as a result of our economic system. Roughly eight million people die each year as a direct consequence of air pollution, and almost as many from pharmaceutical side effects. Little or nothing is reported about this in prominent news outlets—and so much could be done and changed in these areas if the "value of every human life" were really the central motive of political and social action. Where are the "live updates" for the five hundred thousand malaria deaths per year, seventy-five percent of them children, most of which could be prevented and are at least partly the result of the ecological destruction caused by leading industrialized nations? Clemens G. Arvay writes about such connections, which young people should know about and which should become part of general education. Even in Europe there is so much suffering from illnesses that could be prevented. Where is the corresponding media attention with daily statistics and reports from the ICU about the victims of car accidents or socially accepted alcohol consumption?

But back to the socioeconomic situation in a narrower sense and to COVID-19. Various studies have now been published showing the close correlation between the escalation of the disease in many of the so-called "hotspots" with the extent of impoverishment and industrial air pollution, overcrowded living conditions, and poor sanitation. There are a multitude of serious respiratory illnesses, even beyond COVID-19, that develop under these conditions, in these exploited, poverty-stricken parts of the world that have no presence or voice in the media. People's immune systems are severely weakened under the weight of these conditions—not to mention in dreary, under-supplied nursing homes or by incorrect, superfluous antibiotic use or clustered vaccinations. The life expectancy of rich and poor people in Brazil, even beyond COVID-19, differs by no less than eighteen years; but even in Germany the difference is almost ten years. It should be part of general education—even for young people—to know about the various empirical studies on the connection of the human immune system with socioeconomic and sociopsychological living conditions. These include the immunological consequences of unemployment and the role of stress and anxiety in weakening our immunological defenses—of stress and anxiety caused by the socioeconomic situation, by traumatization, and possibly also by media-induced epidemics of anxiety. These facts should, in my opinion, be discussed together with young people and taken seriously; they are aspects of the world in which we live—a world whose problems are much more complex than the leading media coverage of the last months would have us believe. The anthroposophic physician Thomas Hardtmuth wrote in 2020:

> Today one can measure *in time* how our immune system literally collapses when we are chronically humiliated, marginalized, degraded, and not accepted as human beings. When hunger, misery, war, fear, terror, cold, confinement prevail, then diseases and epidemics break out. In the wars of the last centuries, more people have died from cholera, typhus, spotted fever, malaria, etc., than from actual acts of war. This is not only due to pathogens but to the loss of the human sphere of autonomy—when, through fear and terror, we lose our sense of self and thus any motivation to live; there we withdraw from the world and our immune systems collapse.
>
> We also know today that loneliness, which is always accompanied by severe (abandonment) anxiety, is one of the most serious health risk factors. Numerous studies show that the mortality risk from loneliness is higher than from smoking, alcohol, or obesity.... The decline of epidemics and infectious diseases in the nineteenth and twentieth centuries was, contrary to an often-heard claim, not based on medical success through vaccinations and antibiotics, but was almost exclusively due to the improvement of living conditions, such as clean, dry housing, warm clothing, sufficient healthy food, hygiene, clean drinking water, and social stability.[15]

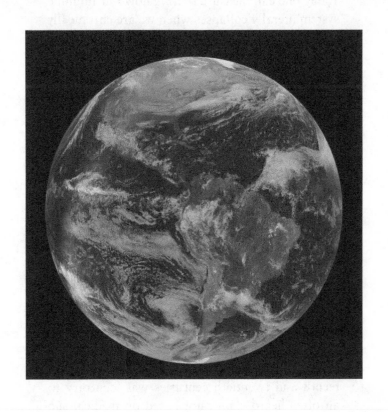

Earth from space
(NASA / NOAA GOES Project)

Consequences of Global Lockdown

To raise the level of discussion about the current situation and overcome easy polarizations, I would also like to consider the global consequences of the Covid measures. Many of us were only marginally affected by them—and quite a few of my acquaintances found the whole thing pleasant for many months: the reflection on family and home in a quieter world, the "deceleration," the relaxing schedule and the end of hectic busyness, the clear skies, the quiet streets, the intense experiences of nature, and also the intensification of individual relationships in the midst of general isolation, the feeling of connectedness and mutual concern, even if often only on the phone, by letter, or virtually on the screen. The question is, however, whether these privileged personal experiences are really sufficient for understanding and assessing the overall situation.

While, as mentioned before, the wealth of the approximately 650 billionaires in the US increased from one trillion dollars to a total of approximately four trillion dollars during the COVID-19 pandemic, countless people worldwide became impoverished on a catastrophic scale, through the loss of all their meager earnings, through the interruption of supply and production chains, through stay-at-home orders that kept them stuck in poor conditions, etc.

The WHO most recently declared that the lockdown measures had caused a "terrible global catastrophe." According to a UN report, the global measures put about 1.6 billion people at risk of losing their livelihoods and 150 million children at risk of acute poverty. Hunger, unemployment, and bankruptcies, as well as medical and psychological illnesses, have reached all-time highs worldwide. Oxfam reported that by July 2020 alone, approximately 121 million more people have been pushed into absolute starvation—and predicts, as a whole, approximately one million additional deaths from hunger in 2020. While people in First World nations spent months anxiously discussing whether or not summer vacations at faraway destinations would be possible and how long they would have to do without major sporting events and parties, the director of the UN's World Food Program spoke of an extreme "hunger pandemic." And while voices that were critical of the rigid lockdown measures could hardly speak out without being socially defamed and ostracized as "Covid deniers," "covidiots," sociopaths, or right-wing extremists, the numbers of victims of other diseases in developing countries increased, in some cases dramatically, especially the deaths among malaria and tuberculosis patients, because attention was centered solely on COVID-19 and because medical examinations and therapies of other diseases were often no longer possible or allowed, combined with a dramatic deterioration of general living conditions. Current estimates are that the additional malaria deaths in Africa will exceed the total number of Covid deaths on the continent by a *factor of ten*. Is it really all about saving human lives? Many thoughtful contemporaries, without being "Covid deniers" or "conspiracy theorists," have asked and continue to ask this in light of these correlations.

However, the need is not only great in Africa, and it seems important to me to broaden the educational horizons of young people to include the suffering that is taking place in their own countries as a result of the Covid measures. The "global consequences of the lockdown" include not least of all the enormous psychological strain on many people, including the mentally ill, sick, old, or dying, who have been deprived of the most precious thing that was left to them in their lives— human relationships and close contact. To my knowledge, the worldwide suicide figures since the beginning of the Covid measures have never been published—and they will probably remain in the dark forever. But it's also not just about suicide from despair due to profound loneliness and isolation. "That I sit the day emotionless, and mute as a child, / Only from my eye often the cold tear still creeps..." as Kermani quoted Hölderlin and his "foreign gaze" in the Homburg speech,[16] also without being a "Covid denier."

Since March 2020, we have experienced the contradiction of a "protection" that can turn into its opposite.

We should develop an awareness of what has been taken away from many people, including hundreds of millions of children, in relation to their schools, their friends, and their daily routines—and realize that the seemingly simple rationale of crisis management does not hold up upon closer examination. The situation is much more complex, and I believe high school classes should also engage this complexity. We must talk about the way society has dealt with the elderly and the sick up to now, and ask ourselves why such nursing homes are so poorly equipped in every respect—in terms of personnel, construction, atmosphere, therapy, soul, and spirit—and how they could ever have arisen in a prosperous industrialized country; these nursing homes already had enormous mortality rates during "normal" flu epidemics.

We must also ask whether the lockdown, in the way it has been implemented, does not permanently weaken many people's immune systems, among them especially the elderly and the sick through the lack of access to nature, light, encounters, and sensory experiences, especially when confined to their room. Where were and are these consequences enumerated and published? How do we arrive at a more differentiated perspective?

Finally, when discussing the consequences of the global lockdown and the other Covid measures, we must also consider and discuss their effects on the sphere of human and civil rights, on the democratic constitutions of many countries. The UN Commissioner for Human Rights, Michelle Bachelet—not a "Covid denier" either—warned of a "human rights catastrophe" on November 23, 2020. Seven months earlier, on April 25–26, 2020, the renowned political journalist and longtime department head of the *Süddeutsche Zeitung*, Heribert Prantl, had already written about this problem, which he by no means sees only in relation to authoritarian states or dictatorships. The political state of emergency was and is, according to Prantl even then, dangerous for the democratic polity, possibly life-threatening, but not only in medical terms. His article was entitled: *"Verfallsdatum? Das Virus als Gesetzgeber: Viele Grundrechtseingriffe werden womöglich auf Dauer bleiben—zur Vorbeugung* [Expiration date? The virus as a legislator: Many encroachments on fundamental rights may remain as a preventive measure—in perpetuity]. I will return to this issue below.

Foreknowledge of the Coming Crisis

Developments in February and March of 2020 happened quickly, and young people were caught by surprise—as we all were. Life was changing rapidly, from day to day, from regulation to regulation, worldwide. All of us were stunned—but it is important to note, I think, that the "measures" as well as the changes in the media and in political, social, and other aspects of life in the wake of the pandemic were not invented in those months. The vast majority of us did not see this crisis coming, did not see it coming in this way—this crisis and these measures. But certain groups of people in leading positions did, perhaps because both the pandemic and the responses to it were, in some respects (e.g., ecologically and virologically), *inherent to the system*, self-inflicted, and to that extent foreseeable. As historical-political studies show, preparations for a dangerous situation, such as the outbreak of a global pandemic, have been in the works for more than twenty years. However, the aim has not been to avert the danger by changing or correcting the system through new values in ecological, socioeconomic, and political terms—or in terms of a "peace policy" with regard to the natural environment—but solely in the sense of system-stabilizing crisis management, combined with far-reaching vaccination strategies. Georg Soldner rightly emphasizes that "this pandemic was foreseeable, but no care was taken";[17] however, a certain "preparation" did take place—a preparation, but no *care*.

In my opinion, these contexts should be part of social studies and contemporary history lessons in high school because they also help, as I see it, to better understand the world in which we live—the world in which children and young people will have to find their way and whose future they will shape. If one takes note of these processes, the overall picture of the crisis becomes more complex, but in some respects also more understandable. It is to Paul Schreyer's great credit that in the summer of 2020, after various publications by individual authors on this subject, he was able to present, on the basis of extensive research, a readable, handy monograph: *Chronik einer angekündigten Krise: Wie ein Virus die Welt verändern konnte* [Chronicle of an announced crisis: How a virus was able to change the world].[18] Many people have now read this study, and I will summarize below a key section from it that deals with the exercise scenarios for a dangerous pandemic outbreak that have been taking place in the US for two decades.

In these staged role-play simulations, international participants implemented measures very similar to the present ones. These included imposing a political state of emergency with extensive restrictions on civil liberties and freedom of movement, targeting public opinion while devaluing alternative viewpoints, even dealing with public unrest on the way to mass vaccination. Schreyer describes in detail how Johns Hopkins University—financed by US billionaires and other private donors—was suddenly omnipresent beginning in March 2020, with daily reports even in the German mainstream media. He also describes how a Center for "Biodefense," later "Biosecurity," and finally "Health Security" was built up beginning at the end of the 1990s in the interplay of a military-industrial and health-political complex, as a "hub of scientific conferences, emergency exercises, and as a means of disseminating the subject to the public through the use of scare tactics. Researchers, military leaders, and politicians met there, and plans and guidelines were developed that soon became influential worldwide."[19] The participants dealt with the challenges of bioweapons and epidemics in, according to Schreyer, a "murky gray area of threat defense and threat generation."[20]

Even after 1997, the CIA had a bacterial bomb developed "of a purely defensive nature."[21] Meetings were held on the subject of pandemics. These meetings revolved around pandemic plans and the necessary crisis management—for example, in the event of a bioweapons attack—and took place in the form of simulation games or exercise scenarios, which from the outset envisaged instilling fear in the population in order to gain political ground for maneuvering. It is "a history that is as long as it is disturbing," according to Paul Schreyer.[22]

As he reports in his research—which he documented with readily accessible sources and which, in my opinion, is no fantastical "conspiracy theory"—the Center's first major conference took place as early as 1999 (now twenty-two years ago) in a Washington, D.C., luxury hotel not far from the Pentagon, and was attended by more than nine hundred participants from ten countries. For two days, the group, consisting of military officers, politicians and bureaucrats, researchers, representatives of lobbying organizations and major pharmaceutical companies, dealt with matters of bioterrorism. New pharmaceutical products, developed in the "interest of national security," played a central role from the beginning and were given top priority. Richard Clarke, the US National Coordinator for Counterterrorism, emphasized at the time:

> For the first time, the Department of Health and Human Services is part of the national security apparatus of the United States....
>
> The current bioterrorism initiative includes a new concept: the first-ever procurement of specialized medicines for a national civilian protection stockpile. As new vaccines and medicines are developed, that program can be expanded. The initiative includes invigoration of research and development in the science of biodefense; it invests in pathogen genome sequencing, new

vaccine research, new therapeutics research, and development of improved detection and diagnostic systems.[23]

Far from being solely in the hands of politicians, however, the project was developed with the significant participation of leading corporations in the health industry, in the form of "global, industrial epidemic management" (Hardtmuth)[24] to be implemented by overstretched national governments in the event of an emergency.

Remarkably, as early as 1999, the question was how to develop a targeted strategy to allow only uniform information to reach the public through media in the event of a threat—and how to deal with the existence of unofficial channels that did not convey the desired view of the threat. ("The question of how to control the message going out to the public was on the minds of all the panelists.")[25] Information presented in the media, it was said, would have to be "coherent and credible," partly in order to be able to achieve a broad or, if possible, complete consensus among the population on the need for vaccination. They also discussed the use of emergency powers and many related questions: "How far can police go to quarantine patients?" "Without a vaccine, the only method of control is isolation, which impedes the spread of the disease but cannot stop it."[26] The pandemic scenario that played out in 1999 was already about the global spread of a disease. The "epidemic response scenarios" of the following year also dealt with the isolation measures that would be applied differently by individual countries in the event of an emergency, with restrictions on freedom of movement in public and with bans on gatherings "of more than a few important people," with the closure of highways, airports, and train stations—but also with the fundamental question of "whether or not this kind of forced isolation and quarantine is a good idea."[27]

According to Schreyer, the 1999/2000 role-play simulations, which dealt with smallpox and the plague, were refined in subsequent years and involved increasingly high-ranking and professional participants. In 2003, the fictional role of the US president was played by former Secretary of State Madeleine Albright and the WHO chief by a former Norwegian prime minister who had herself actually headed the WHO. By 2001, the meeting was no longer held in a hotel but in a highly secured military base near Washington, D.C.— with fewer participants, all of whom held key positions in government agencies, consulting firms, and research institutions. According to Schreyer, in their professional careers they moved "seamlessly between state and private institutions."[28] Starting in 2001, prominent journalists from major media corporations were also invited as observers; in 2005, for example, the US correspondents for *Zeit* and the *Frankfurter Allgemeine Zeitung* participated in the scenario for the first time. Statistics, case figures, and curves were presented, just as they were in reality in 2020. Public life was shut down in the simulation, schools and borders were closed, and the declaration of martial law was considered. Questions of compulsory vaccination and, once again, the suppression of unwanted information were discussed, including possible laws banning "dangerous information."[29] The overcrowding of hospitals was simulated; public unrest due to the pandemic decrees was discussed, as well as the resulting economic and democratic fallout, and much more.

As early as 2001, a "Public-Private Health Partnership" between the WHO and the pharmaceutical industry had been contractually established at the World Economic Forum in Davos; since then, seventy-five percent of funding for the WHO—with its annual budget of approximately four billion dollars—comes from the pharmaceutical industry. In addition, after the attacks of September 11, 2001, transnational structures were created to synchronize policies for national response plans; the concept of "biosecurity" was institutionalized and internationalized. Beginning in 2002, the WHO played an increasingly important role in the Center's simulations at Johns Hopkins University, with the scenarios becoming more complex each year. In 2003, teams from the Robert Koch Institute and the German Ministry of Health participated, as did EU representatives. The simulations were no longer held in one location, but in eight different countries under the title "Global Mercury."

According to Paul Schreyer's analyses, the focus of the scenarios then shifted away from bioterrorism and toward "natural" pandemics starting in 2005, the first of which appears to have been bird flu. Although, according to WHO figures, the bird flu ultimately resulted in only 122 fatalities, it had previously been declared a "world danger" by the US government and mainstream media; Klaus Stöhr, the head of the WHO's influenza program, predicted no fewer than seven million deaths at the time. Nations around the globe purchased billions of dollars' worth of vaccines, and Stöhr ended up transitioning to the pharmaceutical manufacturer Novartis, where, Schreyer says, he remains to this day.

Four years later, the WHO again declared the highest alert level of a "global pandemic" due to swine flu; the German federal government was forced under the Davos Treaty to buy $200 million worth of vaccines from pharmaceutical giant GlaxoSmithKline, the WHO's main funder alongside the Bill and Melinda Gates Foundation. Eighty-one million people were vaccinated in the US, although, as with bird flu, it again turned out to be a costly false alarm; the pharmaceutical industry, however, walked away with eighteen billion dollars in revenue.

In 2010, the Rockefeller Foundation published various future scenarios, including the "Lock-Step" pandemic scenario, which portrayed a future vision of a global authoritarian surveillance state following an influenza epidemic and subsequent economic crisis. China became a global role model in this scenario because of its particularly authoritarian and radical protective measures (including mask mandates). "Even after the pandemic faded, this more authoritarian control and oversight of citizens and their activities stuck and even intensified," this scenario states.[30]

According to Paul Schreyer, the Center for Biosecurity conferences did not take place in their original form after 2005 and were reactivated only after Donald Trump took office and Bill Gates appeared at the World Economic Forum in Davos in January 2017 and at the Munich Security Conference afterward. At Davos, Gates joined with pharmaceutical manufacturers and governments to found the comprehensive vaccine research initiative CEPI (Coalition for Epidemic Preparedness Innovations). In Davos and Munich, he called for more emergency maneuvers to prepare for possible future terrorist-triggered pandemics or even for any "vagaries of nature." An airborne pathogen—via aerosols—could kill more than thirty million people in a year, Gates said. "We need to . . . prepare for epidemics the way the military prepares for war."[31]

Three months later, Schreyer said, extensive planning for a new pandemic exercise took place again for the first time at the "Johns Hopkins Center for Health Security." The fictional focus this time was on a novel viral mixture that had been developed in the laboratory of a biotech company. In this scenario, the terrorist group ABD, "A Brighter Dawn," had set out to slow and eventually reverse global population growth with the viral mixture. Their group members, according to the simulation, had bioscience-virology training—and for the first time, the script included a PCR test to detect the virus. Within this May 2018 exercise in Washington, the production of a vaccine against the viral mixture was expected to take place within months, rather than years—a first for the technologically complex mRNA vaccines, as well.

The final exercise of the entire sequence then took place, according to Schreyer, on October 18, 2019, at a luxury New York hotel ("Event 201") and was optimally staffed with executives from high-profile corporations playing themselves for the first time in the history of the role-play simulations. Participants included the world's largest pharmaceutical company (Johnson and Johnson), the world's largest PR agency, the chief crisis manager of Lufthansa, and also the director of the Chinese Center for Disease Control and Prevention. According to Schreyer, the primary goal was to train governments to cooperate with international corporations and to provide further training for executives; everything was financed by the Gates Foundation and the Davos World Economic Forum, in which the one thousand largest global corporations are united for the close interlocking of corporate and government interests. For the first time, a coronavirus pandemic was now simulated in the exercise; the virus was no longer the result of bioterrorism but was transmitted to humans via bats and pigs. The scenario envisaged that the virus would be easily transmitted to others by people with only mild symptoms, leading to sixty million deaths. The previous themes of the meetings were again present, with a focus on vaccine funding and development; corporations were to play a more active role in politics; targeted PR strategies were to overcome initial resistance among the public. It was a matter—literally—of "trust in science and governments" and of fending off "conspiracy theories" and "conspiracy theorists" who, in the scenario of the exercise, claimed that the pharmaceutical industry itself had been responsible for the spread of the virus.

In contrast, "our side of the story" was to be consistently disseminated.[32] The PR strategy took an internationally centralized approach, which was brought to the public via appropriate representatives. Of paramount importance was the creation of a database as the basis of globally disseminated facts and "key messages." The population needed to be persuaded to change its behavior in the direction "we want to see."[33] Recommendations at the end of the exercise included intensified cooperation between governments and corporations, expansion of international vaccine reserves, dismantling existing vaccine regulations, and a heightened fight against "misinformation":

> Governments will need to partner with traditional and social media companies to research and develop nimble approaches to countering misinformation. This will require developing the ability to flood media with fast, accurate, and

consistent information.... National public health agencies should work in close collaboration with WHO to create the capability to rapidly develop and release consistent health messages. For their part, media companies should commit to ensuring that authoritative messages are prioritized and that false messages are suppressed including though the use of technology.[34]

As Schreyer demonstrates in detail, the 2005 scenario already envisioned the announcement of a smallpox outbreak as the starting point of a global pandemic at the time of a summit meeting of heads of government; the summit then allowed for optimal coordination of further action. This fifteen-year-old simulation suddenly became reality at the World Economic Forum in January 2020, in the presence of corporate giants from the digital and pharmaceutical industries, as well as leading major banks and media representatives. After that, according to Schreyer, the "pandemic machine" to contain SARS-CoV-2 was running under its own steam.

Paul Schreyer's historical documentation is not based on secret documents but on readily available sources; documents about the outlined planning exercises were at least partially publicly available. "Important players have been thinking through the political and social opportunities and challenges created by fear-inducing pandemics for at least ten years," Norbert Häring of *Handelsblatt* magazine also noted.[35] German Health Minister Jens Spahn spoke at a federal press conference on February 27, 2020, saying that plans had already been underway to establish a department for "health security" (that is, biosecurity) in the German Ministry of Health headed by a German army general in late 2019, probably in the aftermath of Event 201.

> We already decided two or three months ago that there will be a new department in the Federal Ministry of Health, a department for health security, because we have noticed in the last few years that this topic—how to prepare for situations like this, and what networks are in place in Europe and internationally—has become more and more important.[36]

The general in charge had previously led a NATO agency for "early diagnosis of infectious disease outbreaks in near-real time" and "centralized surveillance of deployed forces."[37] The US concept of "biosecurity," which unites military, medical-pharmaceutical, and industrial concerns, thus also made its way institutionally into the German Ministry of Health.

Evaluating the events described by Schreyer is not easy. What is certain, however, is that there was advance knowledge of impending epidemics and pandemics, and that sophisticated action plans at the supranational level were rehearsed long before 2020 in the US and its allied states. Furthermore, it is beyond doubt that, from the very beginning, there were also a lot of money and corporate interests at stake; private companies, especially the large-scale vaccine manufacturers, were not only *part* of the scenarios but were among the *organizers* of the meetings. Moreover, it is evident that the political and economic institutions had close ties due to personnel transitions and that the respective interests were difficult to distinguish. It is also clear that, from the beginning, military or military-political goals were involved—"national security interests"—as well as a merging of military and health policy in this area (as evinced, for example, in the creation of a new department of the German Ministry of Health). Finally, Schreyer's chronicle reveals how the "simulations" became increasingly real—until they finally condensed into physical reality.

In his monograph, Paul Schreyer never strays as far from the script of Event 201 as the "conspiracy theorists" who blame the spread of Covid on the profiting pharmaceutical companies themselves. Instead, he holds back entirely on interpretations and merely chronicles the events. What cannot be overlooked, however, is that from the very beginning, experts in various fields—including epidemiology, biological warfare, and zoonotic diseases—were also involved in the conferences, and some of them had themselves been active in related research, in an "opaque gray area of threat defense and threat generation" (Schreyer). It is also certain that the Biodefense or Biosecurity Center did not aim to contribute proactively to the prevention of further zoonoses and pandemics (e.g., by initiating far-reaching change at the ecological and socioeconomic level); rather, the task of the Center was and is to develop response plans for acute crises while maintaining the previous system and its system-immanent "threat generation." This was not a matter of preventive health policy but of reactive "health security" with a military-strategic orientation—"a state of emergency, mass vaccination, and expanded government crackdowns. That was what was being rehearsed" (Schreyer).[38]

It is widely known that preparations—risk analyses and government action plans—for epidemic emergencies have existed not only at the US Center for Biosecurity or Health Security for many years, but also in countries such as South Korea, Taiwan, and Singapore after the SARS epidemic of 2002—and that the German Parliament had a detailed risk analysis prepared in 2012 in the event of a SARS epidemic. Nevertheless, the supranational center in the US that merges military and corporate interests has a special significance—and much of what discerning people have been concerned about since the spring of 2020 has already been rehearsed in these role-play simulations. It also formed part of the aforementioned 2010 Rockefeller Foundation scenario of the future: "Even after the pandemic faded, this more authoritarian control and oversight of citizens and their activities stuck and even intensified." I'll come back to this later.

The Role of the Media

The mass media played a decisive role in the bio-security plans from the very beginning and was responsible for disseminating the desired message and excluding all alternative views. The scenarios were about conveying the same "key messages" over and over again, not allowing anything that deviated from them, and thereby creating effective behavioral norms. ("For their part, media companies should commit to ensuring that authoritative messages are prioritized and that false messages are suppressed, including through the use of technology" [Oct. 20, 2019].)

How many young people have become dubious of the media landscape since February/March 2020? What is needed in order to notice the essential problems of Covid messaging? Looking back on the first months of the Covid crisis, the health ecologist Clemens Arvay—who had worked closely with media representatives in his research and publications in the preceding years—speaks of a "media scandal." In his book *Wir können es besser* [We can do better],[39] he outlines this scandal impressively, but without any exaggeration—indeed, quite soberly: the myriad shocking images and lurid headlines about the deadliness of the pandemic; the tendency toward exaggeration for dramatic effect; the positioning of the "killer virus" as the dominant topic to the exclusion of everything else; the search for the first dead in Germany, which was finally broadcast on March 9 in *Tagesschau* ("The media had literally been eagerly awaiting this event: When, 'finally,' would the first Germans die?");[40] and the horrendous predictions of the expected death toll that were broadcast on all channels. Bill Gates prophesied that up to ten million people would die from COVID-19 in Africa in the foreseeable future, and already by the end of July, eighteen thousand would perish. "Horror scenarios" dominated media coverage of a virus that would never go away or always come back, putting all in mortal danger: "War in the body: This is how Covid kills." Images of coffins in Bergamo or ICUs in New York went around the world in a flash, creating a climate of fear and mass panic among the population and, arguably, among many politicians.

Arvay describes how the images and thoughts of a "killer virus" were still held on to even after it had long since become clear that the lethality of COVID-19 was far below what had originally been indicated—or that the situation in northern Italy, whose special conditions had been researched in the meantime, would not be repeated in Germany in the same way. Arvay speaks of a "misdirection," a will operating within it, and an extraordinary "media pull" that created political compulsion—and vice versa ("...who is pushing whom ahead: the media the politicians, or vice versa... ").[41] In his opinion, the situation in Austria and Germany got completely out of control, not primarily in medical terms but in the media, which made a multifaceted discussion and consideration impossible and weakened people instead of strengthening them—"the strongest pathogenic factor for humankind is chronic, negative, fearful stress" (Hardtmuth).[42] The images dug deep into people's collective memory—including children and adolescents—and were intended to do just that. This also applies to the numbers and statistics presented over and over again, which had many flaws, including the cumulative counting of deaths without reference to population figures and other comparative variables, the grossly simplified and sometimes completely false representations of viruses and the human immune system, and much more.

I wish that every high school—by no means only the Waldorf schools, which I myself did not attend as a child and adolescent—presented the students with a short but sound and differentiated main lesson on the role of the media in the Covid crisis. The lesson would also address the mass media's handling of serious critics, including highly regarded scientists—such as the epidemiologist John Ioannidis of Stanford University— who articulated their concerns early on, warned against the "trap of sensationalism," wanted the possibilities of natural immune defenses against SARS-CoV-2 to be addressed in a more nuanced way, warned of the consequences—including the medical consequences—of the global lockdown, and made a more realistic assessment of the lethality of the virus.

One day, there will be a much more detailed reappraisal of how outsider opinions like those of Ioannidis were handled in the media, how videos—including those of famous epidemiologists—were deleted ("This video has been removed because it violates the YouTube Community Guidelines"), how one form of science or one direction of scientific research and practice was stylized as *the* science and what monopolization and abuse was and is committed in this respect, how other voices than the desired ones were not given any space—not even that of a country like Sweden, which chose a different path and was widely defamed because of it—and how few if any of the many critical articles that appeared in medical journals found their way into the mass media. All this corresponded to the scenarios that had been rehearsed for many years in which the media was given the task of disseminating "key messages" and suppressing other content—whether they concerned the PCR test, infection rates or vaccination, alternative therapeutic approaches for increasing the body's own defenses, or activating treatments or prophylaxis in general (as opposed to mere isolation).

A study of ten million people in China—which is said to have shown in November of this year (2020) that those who tested positive without clinical symptoms are most likely not infectious—was only talked about in alternative channels, obviously because it contradicted the "key message." Only global vaccination would allow for a return to "normalcy," Bill Gates proclaimed on *Fox News*, in accordance with the long-established guidelines, and fear must obviously be maintained until the vaccines can finally save us. Mass media adopted, unchecked, the PR messages of the pharmaceutical industry and embraced completely uncritically, even euphorically, the new genetic vaccine technologies, which were now to be used for the first time and as the "only way out," with a drastic shortening of approval procedures in the rapid "reduction of bureaucracy" (but actually also of safety standards). In his Frankfurt speech on the "pandemic of authoritarianism," Amartya Sen spoke of the "brutal suppression of dissent" in repressively run states, where human rights activists are turned into "terrorists" in a practice that has been successfully implemented for many years. But even in democratically run states, critics of the lockdown and the new vaccine technology—presented as the only option—have been denounced in short order as "covidiots" and "conspiracy theorists," in a flippant take on populist clichés that have suddenly become ubiquitous. In Frankfurt, Sen quoted Immanuel Kant: "The public use of reason must at all times be free, and that alone can bring about enlightenment among human beings."[43]

Critical scientists such as Ioannidis, Wodarg, Streeck, Bhakdi, Arvay, or the Cologne group around

Professor Matthias Schrappe, never denied the existence of Covid or of severe, very severe, and fatal cases, but nevertheless—or precisely because of this—they recommended a different approach. In the media, however, they were completely pushed to the sidelines, although (or because?) Wodarg had been right in 2005 in the discussions about the "global threat" of bird flu.

The American philosopher Charles Eisenstein speaks of the creation of a "war thinking"—an extreme politicization and militant defamation of dissenting views and at the same time an "association of moral virtue with the war effort," which elevates compliance with the Covid measures to the new yardstick of compassion and solidarity.[44] According to Eisenstein, anyone who refuses to completely embrace the claim that Covid is an unprecedented killer virus, or the ban on social contact, or forced masking, is declared to be "antisocial, cynical, or immoral," even though the usefulness of mandatory masks in everyday life continues to be scientifically disputed. Social pressure rather than medical reasoning dominates, and the media plays a large role here. If one wants to understand why a student calls the police because of a maskless teacher, one has to know these contexts.

Against this background, it would also be interesting for high schoolers to read, for example, Stefan Zweig's important 1916 essay "Die Bücher und der Krieg" [Books and war] (from the volume *Worte haben keine Macht mehr: Essays zu Politik und*

Zeitgeschehen [Words no longer have power: Essays on politics and contemporary events], which speaks, among other things, of the "feverish forward race of the image," the "degenerate impatience of curiosity," the "news of the opinions of the hour," and the "rush of events," of an accelerating media machine at the beginning of a wartime inferno in which exaggerations and lies are willingly accepted. Zweig writes, "One walked up and down in one's room, always thinking of it, and yet wanting to think of something else, to be somehow released from this painful hypnosis of time."[45] This was relived by many in 2020.

In the context of the intensified media landscape, the philosopher of education Matthias Burchardt recalled the extensive monograph *The Shock Doctrine: The Rise of Disaster Capitalism* by the Canadian journalist, globalization critic, and climate activist Naomi Klein, which appeared in 2007. Burchardt underlined the need to know about the sociopsychological dynamics of "shock tactics" and their specific "shock doctrines," which—in the sense of the biosecurity scenarios—work with the methods of spreading universal fear and lead to the disorientation of the population by evoking horrendous dangers that are largely removed from their own experience but are conveyed to them by the media. Some of these dangers are real, but others are hypothetical, and the defense against them relies on the advice of a narrow circle of "experts" who are given the status of a single, monolithic authority. According to Burchardt and Klein, this provides a means of enforcing political decisions by exerting tremendous social pressure on the population to accept the decisions as the only possible solution, even though they bypass the participation of civil society and are implemented through a top-down emergency system.

Klein's theses and her historical examples of the effectiveness of "shock tactics" are controversial in the secondary literature, but they are worth taking hold of and discussing in high school in light of the events of 2020 and our own entanglement in these issues. Young people are capable of doing this—as long as they are not "left alone." The analyses of Rainer Mausfeld, emeritus professor of psychology at the University of Kiel, which are distinctly critical of the media, are, in my opinion, of interest in this context, and excerpts could be worked with in high school.[46]

Mausfeld describes how, in order to maintain its neoliberal order of domination and de facto violence, the Western world rooted in "shared values" selectively uses the mass media for the purpose of directing consciousness—with destructive consequences in "exploited" emerging countries, but also in the "West" itself. According to Mausfeld, the mass media stabilizes the social and economic status of those who own or fund it; furthermore, it not only stabilizes existing power structures but also enables the broad acceptance of measures that would not gain majority support without a targeted selection and interpretation of facts, without an enhancement and manipulation of images, indeed without mass media "opinion and dissent management," which Mausfeld explains using the example of various wars of aggression in the guise of "humanitarian interventions" or the financial "rescue" of Greece by the EU and IMF. He speaks of a manipulation of attention and emotion that has long since replaced old dictatorial control techniques and is effective as an invisible ideology and unquestioned framework—while maintaining illusions of freedom, co-determination, and democracy. In critical decision-making situations, the aim is a militant conformity that determines what is "unambiguously right," does not allow for complexity and diversity, has a minimal tolerance for ambiguity—in the face of the ambiguity of the situation or problem—and necessarily leads to social polarization, to *divide et impera*, divide and conquer. According to Mausfeld, the mass media is not only involved in this overall process but enables it to proceed at a crucial point.

The question of media impact, selection, and emphasis can be discussed with high school students in this sense, using the example of Covid reporting, provided they are not ideologically fixed and already radicalized or traumatized—and it leads further, in my opinion, to questions of situational- *and* self-knowledge. In such studies, we notice what media reporting does to us—what concrete, real, and personal perception and experience we have and where we merely follow widespread perceptions, judgments, and images, most often completely uncritically.

These books by Mausfeld and Naomi Klein were written before the Covid crisis; there can be no question of them being partisan books on the extremely emotionally charged subject we are now examining. Therefore, one can freely discuss with young people the question of whether their analyses are helpful for a deeper understanding of the current situation, also against the background of the role of the media in the biosecurity pandemic scenarios, as documented by Paul Schreyer.

I also find this topic extremely useful, because young people today are well aware of photograph and video manipulation. They have grown up knowing about "doctored photos," fake profiles, and "social bots," and many of them know—through figures like Sascha Lobo and Edward Snowden—about the manipulability of the internet, which began decades ago as a free and communal medium of communication but, through the influence of high-profile corporations and lobbyists, has long since become something quite different. At least some of them are aware of the illusory freedom of the internet and the economic interests at work in it, including the reality of censorship in so-called "social media"—where it is not the government but large internet corporations that remove alternative viewpoints and enact a "blanket suppression of the undesirable" (Schreyer).[47] Edward Snowden speaks with Shoshana Zuboff about "surveillance capitalism"—and even Clemens Arvay recently had to experience with astonishment that his factually informative video about the problem of shortened vaccine trials was deleted.

Individual young people, at least, are also aware of the dynamics of social environments that promote self-assurance and self-affirmation—the "echo chambers of the internet"—even the ideological constructs of polarized and often fundamentalist groups. Charles Eisenstein wrote about such "communities" "subjecting any contradicting information to hostile scrutiny, [while] each accepts with little question anything that reinforces its own position." This group phenomenon ("groupthink") is readily observable in the controversies surrounding the Covid crisis.[48] Bans on contact and assembly, which drive all social discourse onto the internet, undoubtedly also exacerbate this problem.

The "truth crisis of the digital age" has now become apparent to many young people, also through painful personal experiences on social media. But many of them are left alone with it. Where is the place to reflect on this together, and what is to be done in view of the growing lack of experientiality in a world of almost perfect simulation, in which a person's "appearance" not only precedes reality but can virtually replace it?

"It is already a fact of online life that one's friendly online conversational partner or sensitive online therapist may in reality be only a chatbot.... Other robots…provide 'emotional and social support for older people with dementia,'" writes Thomas Fuchs.[49]

Artificial programs can already take the place of real relationship experiences:

> If a cuddly robot called "Smart Toy Monkey" is supposed to serve as a friend to small children and thereby promote "social-emotional development"; if friendly nursing robots replace the human care of dementia patients and supposedly listen to their stories; or if patients are prescribed programmed online psychotherapies that save them having to see a therapist—then machines become "relationship artifacts," as Sherry Turkle (2011) puts it. (Fuchs)[50]

Of course, the last point is no longer directly related to the Covid problem, but it is related to the world in which we increasingly live and which will be the future world of our young people today. They will have to find their way in this world with a sense of authenticity and genuineness, of mutuality and reciprocity, of real relationships. The problem of a purely virtual existence started to become clear to many young people during the crisis of 2020—the essential difference between their own perceptions and those brought to them by the media, between a real encounter and one that is only virtual or is even an "encounter" with "relationship artifacts." Never before has there been such a dramatic shift of social activities and interactions into virtual space as during the lockdown, even among young people. Their media experiences can therefore form a training ground, but they must also be discussed, reflected upon, and advanced further in the classroom. It is about nothing less than the formation of a new, yet-to-be-refined "sense organ" for *authenticity*. This, too, belongs to the qualitative "right to education" and the standard for evaluating real education—also with regard to tendentious news reports, such as those appearing in *Der Spiegel (online)*.

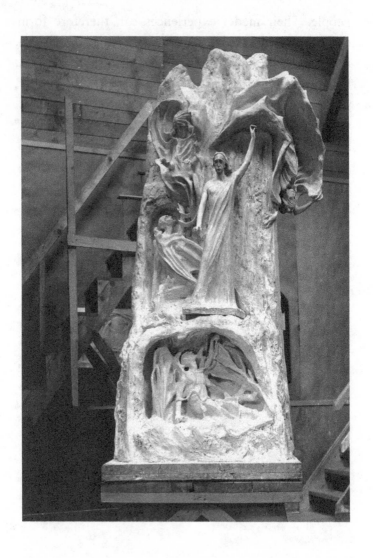

*Model, plaster cast, Edith Maryon and Rudolf Steiner,
ca. 1915/1916 (from Mirela Faldey / David Hornemann v.
Laer, eds., Im Spannungsfeld von Weltenkräften [In the field
of tension between world forces], Dornach, 2020, p. 61)*

Technology and the Image of the Human Being

What should also be explored in the classroom in this context, in my opinion, is the whole question of humanity's belief in technology—the technocratic tunnel vision for the supposed solution of all of society's problems (problems that technical materialism has largely created itself), from climate breakdown to zoonoses; also, the whole problem of the technological imperative, according to which all technical options must be implemented and used. In this context, I think it is also important to discuss with young people the Covid-triggered tendency toward rapid and relentless digitalization, including so-called "digital learning," which lacks real interpersonal dialogue and empathic resonance from a counterpart. It is important to reflect and discuss together whether real "learning" is taking place here at all or merely a step-by-step sequence of information assimilation, processing, and application, a training of desired responses and corresponding behavior.

I recently read in a publication with a critical stance on this subject that the Center for Teacher Education in Cologne claimed that robots are better able to teach than humans due to their "neutrality." In the "neutral" environment they create, it is easier for students to "say something wrong" without being afraid.[51] The argument reminded me of the rationale once used to introduce, or rather impose, the fatal "multiple-choice" examination into the medical education system—with the promise of "equal opportunities" for all due to the absence of a personal counterpart. The "self-abolition of the human being" evident in these examples found an excellent breeding ground in the Covid crisis. I also read that the German Minister of Education and Research, Anja Karliczek, is reported to have said, "The Covid crisis offers Germany a great opportunity in terms of digital education: We can create a real change in mentality. We see how useful digital learning opportunities can be. Everyone is now willing to just give it a try. I see a new mindset awakening."[52]

In my opinion, it is important for young people to think about what kind of "awakening" this really entails and what directions and intentions for the future are asserting themselves here—more effectively than ever before. Ultimately, it is necessary to reflect on whether this is not actually about a struggle for the image of the human being and the future of humanity. The Heidelberg psychiatry professor and outstanding medical anthropologist Thomas Fuchs has recently published the important book *Die Verteidigung des Menschen* [Defending the human being], which is exceedingly relevant for high school students. As the motto of his preface, Fuchs chose a statement by Karl Jaspers: "The image of the human being that we hold to be true becomes itself a factor in our lives."[53] We can ask the students (and ourselves) what "image of the human being" is behind a completely digitalized society; and we can also ask what image of the human being guides a society that retreats from one another into repeated lockdowns.

Matthias Burchardt speaks of "Homo hygienicus," and his work can also be discussed with young people.[54] Where is society heading, and how do young people understand themselves? Do they want the predictable, transparent, controllable, and manageable human being and a society based on such an image of the human being? I do not mean this rhetorically or suggestively—and I am personally sure that alert young people of our time have already had some experience with this problem, and long *before* the Covid crisis. Many of them have experienced what it means to find themselves on the internet as predictable and calculable consumers whose "patterns" have been recorded and processed in order to generate predictions about them. Perhaps you may have heard about the future project of "Anticipatory Shipping," which Amazon has patented. Amazon wants to have products delivered that have not been ordered but are very likely to be of interest based on pre-existing patterns. So far, it just says, "Customers who bought this also bought...." But the algorithmic analysis of customer data and search history has been happening for some time, and not all young people are comfortable with it. Perhaps some suspect that this is not about developing into the future but about holding on to the past and reinforcing what exists, about reproducing what has been ascertained on the basis of "patterns," about being calculated, defined, and fixed; but perhaps it is about much more—namely, about controlling people on the basis of what is known about them. This control will then not be carried out by a dictator and his political party but by the algorithms of the digitalized world, which in the future will very likely not only present product suggestions but also generate decisions in their own way, anonymously and mechanically. The students' vague intuitions about these things could be raised to consciousness in class discussion.

Young people today might also have heard of the Chinese "social credit" model, which has been operating for three years now as a socio-technological system to control human behavior, working through the widespread use of facial recognition software in public spaces. The goal is to condition a "happy society."

Sascha Lobo wrote in his 2019 book *Realitätsschoc* [Reality shock]—which is also suitable for high school students—of the "digitally enabled authoritarianism" of the Chinese model, which he sees as an attractive "export" to Western democracies—a "combination of dictatorship and economic growth, made possible by a radically digital orientation without regard for the loss of fundamental rights."[55] Lobo's work gained heightened poignancy in 2020, when China became a model in the fight against Covid (with a "secure lockdown" and electronic surveillance of potential dangers, especially human "dangers") and when, in the spring of 2020, for the first time, China equaled America in popularity in a German poll. "No country in the world has so aggressively and successfully advanced globalization, then digitization, and now artificial intelligence," Lobo emphasized in 2019,[56] describing in detail the vision of a "cybernetic society" being pursued in China.

> The basis of today's cybernetic ideologies is the constant surveillance of society, the recognition of patterns with the help of the generated data, and the control of behavior on this foundation.[57]

By no means, Lobo continues, is this merely about eliminating political resistance. It is about so much more. Every behavior—including thoughts—is to be recorded, measured, and evaluated in order to be able to control society. Already in 2019, even before the global crisis, Lobo also described tendencies in Western industrialized countries to proceed more and more in this direction—on the basis of economic and "security" interests:

> In two provinces in Canada, a system called RTD (Risk-driven Tracking Database) has been in place for several years. In this system, data from the police, health authorities, the youth welfare office, and other agencies are combined, including speculation about mental illness, substance abuse, and

"antisocial behavior." In this way, risk scenarios are calculated for entire neighborhoods, as well as for specific families and individuals.[58]

The public sphere is becoming "a more and more intensely controlled space" in Europe as well—and with the consent of the population. "A representative survey in spring 2018 in Berlin shows that seventy-five percent of Berliners would like to see more video surveillance," for the purpose of risk avoidance.[59] "The fact that European countries are not yet as radical as China in terms of the surveillance and analysis of the population is due more to inferior technology, resistance from civil society, and the socially liberal side of politics than to a lack of desire on the part of the authorities. The weakening of fundamental rights follows technological capabilities somewhat more slowly in the West, as well."[60]

"The image of the human being that we hold to be true becomes itself a factor in our lives," Karl Jaspers emphasized, and we can and should ask ourselves—and also high school students—what kind of image of the human being is actually at work in this vision of the future. It is certainly not the image of ethical individualism, of the self-responsible, free, and mature individuality who shapes society. The historian and bestselling author Yuval Noah Harari points clearly in the intended direction:

> People will no longer see themselves as autonomous beings running their lives according to their wishes but instead will become accustomed

to seeing themselves as a collection of biochemical mechanisms that is constantly monitored and guided by a network of electronic algorithms.[61]

For Harari, however, this is not a vision of horror but makes a certain sense because "organisms are algorithms. Every animal—including Homo sapiens—is an assemblage of organic algorithms shaped by natural selection over millions of years of evolution."[62] "The single authentic self is as real as the eternal Christian soul, Santa Claus, and the Easter Bunny."[63]

At this point, the basic assumptions of the Chinese model must be urgently questioned—and it is good, sensible, and necessary, I believe, to allow adolescents to do so, or at least to begin to do so. The materialist notion of the unfree human being—as a "collection of biochemical mechanisms constantly monitored and directed by a network of electronic algorithms"—and the creation of the "technology of an unfree world" are closely—indeed, indissolubly—linked. The aim is for people to affirm this world as the "healthiest" and "safest," most efficient and rational, the "best possible world," a world, moreover, that offers the prospect of their own technological "optimization"—not only in regard to upgrading their immune systems to defend against external threats through the most modern forms of genetic engineering, but also in the area of their mental abilities and performance ("enhancement"), their physical appearance and "fitness," their selected modes of reproduction and the arresting of the aging process.

Human beings, thought of as analogous to technical systems, are to be technologically improved:

> With optimized genomes and bodies enhanced by links to external technology, people could be more beautiful...more intelligent, more emotionally sophisticated, more physically able, more socially connected, generally healthier, and happier all round.[64]

The direct transfer of software content to the human brain ("the vision is that in the distant future it will be possible to transfer skills from an app store to the brain via a chip—for example, the movements from martial arts or a new foreign language"[65]) and vice versa is envisaged by "Neuralink systems" ("mind uploading"), up to and including "digital immortality," by which the content of the human brain is copied to other "hardware" and is thought to continue to exist in this way.

What many people still consider futuristic science fiction—the "transhuman" or "posthuman" fantasies of maniacal technologists—has long been advancing in practice, with billions in assets. In the spring of 2020, we were able to see some of the Canadian multi-billionaire Elon Musk's roughly four hundred satellites in the airplane-free night sky. Musk and his company Space X's forty thousand private satellites are soon to orbit the earth for optimum broadband internet coverage. On the other hand, his company Neuralink, which aims to network and ultimately merge the human brain with machines and which gained some momentum four years ago, is still lesser known to the general public (unlike Tesla and PayPal). Thomas Fuchs writes in his book *In Defense of the Human Being*:

> Humanism in the ethical sense therefore means resistance to the rule and constraints of technocratic systems as well as to the self-reification and mechanization of humans. If we conceive of ourselves as objects, be it as algorithms or as neuronally determined apparatuses, then we surrender ourselves to the rule of those who seek to manipulate such apparatuses and to control them socio-technologically. "For the power of Man to make himself what he pleases means...the power of some men to make other men what *they* please." (Lewis)[66]

Economization and Surveillance

There is yet another theme I believe could help to raise the level of the argument and bring to general awareness what is very likely at stake in the current disputes. It seems important to me that young people learn to see through simplifications and schematizations in the media and to question emphasis. Which danger is presented, which is not? What is left out of the daily news speaks volumes when it is noticed. This allows us to think in the direction of the real questions and challenges.

There is much to suggest that what is currently at stake is not only the defense against infectious disease threats of "national scope," but also the central values of society. Young people—and all of us—have witnessed the farewell to culture in the neoliberal materialism of 2020, when everything that was not considered "systemically relevant"—including theaters, museums, and concert halls—was forced to close. I imagine you have a sense of the power of global capitalism, and perhaps you are not surprised by the tremendous profits of the leading billionaire class during the Covid crisis, which is not accidental after all. You are not a "conspiracy theorist" if you begin to ask questions about the workings and effects of the global financial system and about the restructuring underway there, which Klaus Schwab and Thierry Malleret of the World Economic Forum wrote about in a decidedly instructive book in the summer of 2020.[67] Rudolf Steiner warned early on that in the future governments would become "economic bodies in the guise of government bodies" if there were no fundamental reorganization of society in the sense of "social threefolding." Such a future would involve an automatization of spiritual-cultural life (including educational institutions) vis-à-vis the legal and economic realms. "Today it is objective capital that works over the Earth," said Steiner already on March 22, 1919, in Dornach, and he spoke of the "economic interests of capital-imperialism."[68]

In my opinion, our present and near future financial system should be carefully considered in high school—of course, not in all its details but in the sense of an urgently needed democratization of knowledge and an informed questioning. The power of economics has conquered and alienated more and more areas; it is not only ecosystems that have suffered severe and partly irrevocable damage from this campaign of conquest, but also health care systems. Hospitals have fallen into the hands of private, profit-driven investors in recent decades, resulting in the increased industrialization of hospital operations and the "rationalizing away" of large parts of the nursing sector—a fact that is reported at most in passing, even against the backdrop of caring for

Covid-19 patients. I recommend here reading the publications of the Freiburg medical ethicist and internist Giovanni Maio—in particular, the book *Geschäftsmodell Gesundheit: Wie der Markt die Heilkunst abschafft* [The health business model: How the market is abolishing the art of healing], which I also consider suitable material for high school students. It opens one's eyes to a problem that existed many years before Covid-19 and is "inherent in the system." Almost all of the pharmaceutical, hospital, medical device, and "health management" industries are now privately owned. "How can society hope for this industry to be an honest 'partner' in preventing disease?" asks Paul Schreyer.[69] And physician Thomas Hardtmuth adds elsewhere:

> Just as an arms industry has no interest in peace and has fueled many military escalations by financing "rebels" and "insurgents," so the global business in vaccines and antiviral drugs must be animated by ever-new strategies of fearmongering.[70]

The economization of health, including epidemic infectious diseases, and the integration of the health care system into a cybernetic model of societal control are generating an enormous problem. People who draw attention to this today are therefore not "Covid deniers" or "sociopaths," but alert contemporaries. (This social "alertness," it should be noted, was already something that Rudolf Steiner saw as vital to Waldorf high school lessons.)

In the third Civil Protection Act—as an amendment to the Protection against Infection Act—the German Parliament recently authorized the Robert Koch Institute to monitor citizens virologically and in terms of health, granting the Federal Minister of Health far-reaching powers. Edward Snowden, who is also a household name for many young people, was not the only one to warn that the Covid crisis could be used to permanently expand surveillance; in his widely read 2019 autobiography, Snowden described the transition from targeted surveillance of individuals to mass surveillance of entire populations, which he experienced firsthand as an employee in US intelligence agencies.

In an April 2020 report from China, a ZDF television correspondent remarked:

> What frightened me the most, and this is perhaps also a topic that German viewers are very interested in, is how quickly the surveillance state became visible. For every move you want to make, you have to download an app.... People's fear of illness is used to allow this massive surveillance to take place.... Most of the Chinese people we talked to think it's great. The fear of a new wave of infections, a fear that is also guided by the state, is so great that they do not see a restriction of their freedom but something positive that protects them.[71]

In the weeks and months that followed, however, the majority of Germans were obviously no longer concerned about corresponding developments in their own country. Sascha Lobo's prophecy that the Chinese model would become a "top export" seems to have come true faster than expected during the Covid crisis.

Paul Schreyer and others have comprehensively documented that the vision of a total digital record of humanity has already been alive for many years in leading corporate and political circles—for planning and controlling human development, including medicine and population dynamics, especially as regards the long-lamented "overpopulation" of the Earth, which is to be "regulated." "Digital identity"—the individual biometric recording of each person's vaccination status along with other data, down to their molecular makeup—is planned as part of a universal health information system, and "epidemonnomics"* is introduced as a new discipline, with new terminology.

Schreyer and others report on the presentation of a corresponding test model at the Davos World Economic Forum in January 2020, financed by the Rockefeller Foundation, Microsoft, and the "vaccine alliance"—which Bill Gates helped to establish—between pharmaceutical companies, governments, the World Bank, and the WHO. By early 2020, Bangladesh had

---

* Epidemonnomics is a new hybrid discipline that combines molecular epidemiology with population demographics and global economics. See "An Optimist's View of Global Health Achievement: Remarks by Tim Evans, Dean, Bangladesh Rural Advancement Committee (BRAC) University," The Rockefeller Foundation, Feb. 25, 2013, https://www.rockefellerfoundation .org/news/an-optimists-view-of-global-health-achievement/.

already succeeded in capturing the digital biometric data of more than one hundred million people and linking it to other information, including their vaccination status ("ID 2020"). The goal, however, according to Schreyer, is the overall registration of "global citizens," the central storage of their data by giant US corporations with cloud services (such as Amazon and Microsoft). If cash were to be abolished and only digital account transactions were allowed by entering one's digital ID, the surveillance and control possibilities would be nearly limitless.

The state of emergency brought on by the "Covid crisis" accelerates all these developments in a breathtaking way. Knowing about this is part of the "general education" of today, to which everyone has a democratically guaranteed "right."

≈

I now come to the last part of my remarks. I said at the outset that, in my opinion, what is needed among young people is more knowledge and awareness of the problems, and the development of skills that serve to shape the future and overcome crises so that—unlike in Navid Kermani's prophecy—Earth's future can be "saved" after all and not just "endured." So far, I have sketched some of the problems that seem to me to come into question. Now, however, I shall discuss the "skills that serve to shape the future and overcome crises."

DIE

PHILOSOPHIE DER FREIHEIT.

GRUNDZÜGE

EINER

MODERNEN WELTANSCHAUUNG.

VON

DR. RUDOLF STEINER.

Beobachtungs-Resultate nach natur-
wissenschaftlicher Methode.

BERLIN,

VERLAG VON EMIL FELBER.

1894.

*Rudolf Steiner, Die Philosophie der Freiheit
[The Philosophy of Freedom], Berlin 1894*

The *"Inner Concept of Truth"*

I would like to mention first of all the promotion of individual insight and judgment, the promotion of a "sense of truth," as a concrete faculty. I would like to remind you that Rudolf Steiner explicitly wrote this on the banner of the Waldorf School's high school lessons. It is about the formation of a "correct inner concept of truth," which must become a factor of the sovereignty and maturity of the individual. There are sufficient opportunities for this today. The goal, however, is not to find and name *the* supposed culprit or *the* problem in a situation that is challenging to grasp in its entirety, but to examine the various forces that endanger the future of humanity and the Earth. The goal is to endure inconsistencies in news reports and in one's own perceptions, to learn to develop a flexibility of perspective, to recognize tacitly presupposed but nevertheless effective paradigms and to endure ambiguities, even if this is not so easy. "The truth will set you free."

Truth, however, is not a simple and unambiguous fact—at least not in the subject we are talking about—but a complex entity with many sides that must be recognized, endured, and acknowledged. There is nothing paralyzing about this admission; rather, dealing with this complex reality generates an experience of freedom. This conscious experience of freedom helps in the fight against the "pandemic of authoritarianism" (Amartya Sen), and at the same time forms for young people a lasting experience of self. One knows oneself by experiencing oneself as a thinking, reflecting, and discerning human being, as a thinking soul that emancipates itself from dogmas and labels—including those of the mainstream media—and develops trust in its own perceptions and experiences, in its impressions and sensations, on the way to its own "sense of truth."

As Thomas Fuchs states in his book *In Defense of the Human Being*, the difference between human intelligence and so-called "artificial intelligence" (AI)—which wants to leave the "limitations of human cognition" behind (Lobo)[72]—lies in intentional consciousness and in human goal-oriented knowledge, in our capacity for self-experience and self-awareness, in our ability to view and understand our own situation and our own actions from a higher perspective. In contrast to "artificial intelligence," which, according to Fuchs, is alien to real intelligence, human cognition has nothing to do with learning through programs of "pattern recognition," with an algorithmic automation that lacks any orientation toward the future and any actual decision-making ability; rather, human cognition is about self-reflection and self-transcendence. Young people are capable of the latter—or else it is the task of the school to assist them in the development of these abilities.

Anyone who, like me, has seen an outstanding twelfth-grade staging of *Brave New World* knows what today's young people are capable of, what insight into their situation and the situation of the world these young people are capable of—and not only as protagonists on the stage. Aldous Huxley's novel, published in 1932, is about a future society, in the year 2540, in which "stability, peace, and freedom" are apparently guaranteed. Diseases no longer exist in this fictional society; they are eradicated by prenatal vaccinations. People are always healthy and efficient, and aging happens almost imperceptibly. They feel no decline in physical performance and, thanks to exercise and modern cosmetics, they change only slightly externally, even though their lifespan is limited to an age between sixty and seventy. Until then, they remain vital and then die very quickly and painlessly in a "soma" half-sleep. Fear of death is eliminated through conditioning by taking groups of children through hospices where sleeping people can be seen quietly dying.

In order to oppose Huxley's vision or prediction—which can still be considerably elaborated and differentiated in the age of AI and robotics, of chatbots and virtual worlds, of global recording and surveillance, of Space X and Neuralink—young people need forces of enlightenment (in Kant's sense of the word), they need the courage to make use of their own insight. But they also need help in "defending the human being" and their own humanity, in order to see through the seductions of artificial and technological images of the human being—and thus of the self—which, in the sense of Harari, want to make them believe that there is no individual "I" any more than there is a Santa Claus or an Easter Bunny, that they themselves consist only of a "collection of biochemical mechanisms" that are "constantly monitored and guided by a network of electronic algorithms" and cannot be distinguished from computers—even though they may function more slowly and more erroneously.

"Today, hardly anything is more socially urgent than global resistance against the increasing authoritarianism all over the world," said Amartya Sen in October 2020 as he accepted the Peace Prize of the German Book Trade in Frankfurt's St. Paul's Church.[73] But this "authoritarianism" is by no means exercised only by political rulers and dictatorial governments, but also by the paradigmatic determinations of modern materialism and its technology, by its ideological construct of the unfree and undiscerning human being who is to be monitored and controlled. The image of the human being that we hold to be true becomes, according to Jaspers, a "factor" of our life—indeed, it becomes the determining factor of our life.

For many young people, the crises of 2020 involved a painful awakening, a disintegration of sustaining friendships and communities that had previously functioned in a natural way. Because of the lack of contact and because of the different assessments of the Covid situation, there were vehement disputes and fractures, also between young people themselves. Many found themselves turning radically inward, introspectively, more than ever before in their lives. Many grew tired of the virtual world, of online communication, even of media overload. At least some of them struggled to find their own deeply experienced assessment of the truth of the situation and of their personal behavior, tested themselves and reality again and again, and went through amazing developments in difficult times.

Dialogue

I now come to another point. In addition to reflecting on oneself and on the global situation—on the state of humanity and on the image of the human being—which must be done in adolescence, I believe that today more than ever it is a question of developing the capacity for dialogue. The aforementioned disputes over the assessment of the Covid situation—intensified by a comprehensive wave of fear and exacerbated by polarizing portrayals in the mainstream media and the large-scale defamation of critical voices—have led to dramatic cracks and fissures in the social fabric of communities, also in the social fabric of schools and, as previously indicated, even in the lives of young people. Friendships were broken as a result of differing assessments of the situation, its threat level and the measures used to contain it, the ethics and morals demanded by the situation—to an extent previously unknown in the short lifetime of these young people, as conversations with them often reveal. How does one overcome this serious fragmentation?

In my opinion, it is a matter of practicing dialogue with those who are completely different. Young people are capable of this, but they also have to be encouraged to take it up. In the section "Personal Making Present" in his essay "Elements of the Interhuman," Martin Buber wrote, in 1953, about the adult world:

> By far the greater part of what is today called conversation among [people] would be more properly and precisely described as speechifying. In general, people do not really speak to one another, but each, although turned to the other, really speaks to a fictitious court of appeal whose life consists of nothing but listening to him.[74]

Real conversation, Buber continues, is based on the assumption that everyone really, meaningfully regards his or her partner as a concrete person. It is a matter of "becoming aware" of the other in his or her essential otherness and unique perception and conception of the world, in acceptance of how the other is, in respect for the particular inner world "out of which his conviction has grown." Thus, in spite of all the differences of opinion, it is about the acceptance of the other as a *Thou* and about the readiness for a real conversation with one another, even if under difficult conditions:

> Perhaps from time to time I must offer strict opposition to his view about the subject of our conversation. But I accept this person, the personal bearer of a conviction, in his definite being out of which his conviction has grown—even though I must try to show, bit by bit, the wrongness of this very conviction. I affirm the person I struggle with: I struggle with him as his partner,

I confirm him as creature and as creation, I confirm him who is opposed to me as him who is over against me.[75]

Buber would certainly have advised against applying these formulations to a one-to-one conversation between adolescents about the Covid crisis and its various facets. I think he would probably not have wanted young people to engage in "struggle with a partner," but rather to have a real conversation first, an honest exchange about the many perceptions and perspectives each of them has. But, in any case, he would have insisted upon the necessity of a genuine dialogue, in the "reciprocity that has become language," and, if necessary, also the "struggle with a partner." The current social situation demonstrates the need for his approach.

It is more necessary than ever, in the Covid era, to alleviate the "pathological distrust of all against all," to overcome that "xenophobia" which Stefan Zweig describes in his memoirs as the "spiritual epidemic of the twentieth century." If the other human being is seen primarily as a potentially deadly carrier of germs—or as a carrier of irrational, "covidiotic" views that hinder the systematic containment of the virus and thus endanger the general public and each individual—then society ceases to be society; it splinters and disintegrates, it militarizes, and it will again try to remove all dissenting opinions or all dissenting people from its monopolized center, because they are seen as vital threats. The sociologist Stephan Lessenich recently described the "dynamics of excluding people from spaces of legitimacy" within democracy—"outsiders are not always on the outside to begin with, but they are made so at concrete historical moments under concrete social conditions."[76] At least in regard to the community of young people, I believe that the promotion of differentiated thinking and complex, multi-layered situational awareness—as well as genuine dialogue in the sense of Martin Buber—can counteract this process of exclusion. I said at the beginning that it is a matter of raising the qualitative level of the current discussions—both in terms of content, by including broader perspectives, but also in terms of the manner and quality of the exchange. Perhaps the latter is the most important thing of all.

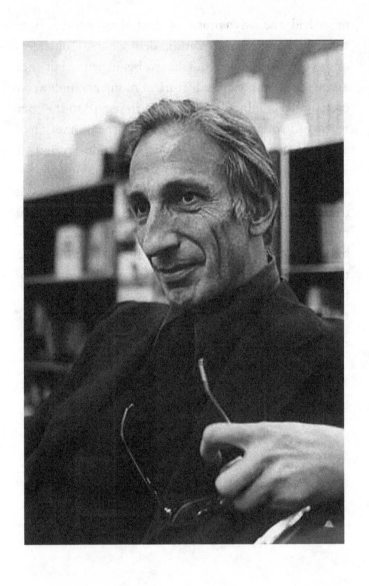

Ivan Illich (1926, Vienna – 2002, Bremen)

Individuality and Immunity

I van Illich emphasized many decades ago:

> Health levels will be at their optimum when the environment brings out autonomous personal, responsible coping ability. Health levels can only decline when survival comes to depend beyond a certain point on the heteronomous (other-directed) regulation of the organism's homeostasis. Beyond a critical level of intensity, institutional health care—no matter if it takes the form of cure, prevention, or environmental engineering—is equivalent to systematic health denial.[77]

Among the skills that should at least be introduced during adolescence, I would also include managing one's own individual health, what Illich calls an "autonomous personal, responsible coping ability" and an "organic balance." The inner life of adolescents and their ability to manage the challenges of life are known to be dynamic and subject to crisis. This is simply part of the structure and processes of this age group. Nevertheless, the self-aware adolescent can also learn to experience his or her "I"-presence in the bodily structure. External "hygiene" is not the only important factor for maintaining one's own immunity and health, but also, for example, "hygienic eurythmy" and many other activities that promote one's own being-at-home in the body and, with this body, in the world. "Only if we inhabit our bodies will we also be able to maintain the Earth in a habitable form," writes Thomas Fuchs.[78]

Among the lessons of the Covid crisis, as outlined above, is the existential importance of ecology and our co-responsibility for it, which begins with caring for our own bodies as part of the Earth. Inescapably pushed into the virtual space in 2020, we were able to experience anew, and learn to experience more consciously, the intrinsic meaning of concrete corporeality, of our own "being incarnate," but also of embodiment in the social space. This holds true for young people as well. The bodily encounter was newly appreciated in its uniqueness and intrinsic value under conditions of increased electronic mediation, also as the "starting and ending point" of the virtual encounter, as Thomas Fuchs notes. The bodily interaction with others shone brightly in 2020 in its indispensability—the "virtual appearance of the other" does not replace real life. The exceptional Covid time, understood in this way, could be experienced not only as a training in sensitivity for embodied presence in the social realm but also as a training in one's own bodily presence—as a prerequisite for directing our attention to the world through the corporeal instrument.

The "I"-presence in the body is a characteristic and decisive factor of human immunity, as Thomas Hardtmuth points out—and it has to do, in turn, with what Christoph Hueck brings to the concept of biographical health. As Hueck explains:

> What we need in place of the ideology of control is more trust in the spiritual powers of the individual, in one's own inner health forces, trust in life in all its facets, trust in reality. Far more than before, we must ask how we can strengthen the inner forces of the human being, because these forces are the real source of health. True, biographical health comes not from external control and avoidance but from inner strength.[79]

Quite a few young people report that after the initial shock and total fear at the beginning of the Covid period, they have slowly found their way back to themselves, to their inner spiritual forces, their autonomous way of coping with life, which no one can take from them but which they also do not want anyone to take from them. In some cases, the crisis was able to lead to growth and maturation on the level of the "I," to a strengthening of the power of the individual in the body and with the body, to an increase of autonomy, possibly also of one's own immunity through activity, through meaningful deeds—both in the outer world and in the inner space of the soul, in creative thinking, feeling, and willing. To work with this kind of self-reflection in the classroom seems to me to be imperative.

A meditative verse from Rudolf Steiner, with which Ita Wegman concluded her daily spiritual work with her Arlesheim Clinic nurses, reads:

> Find yourself in the light
> With the soul's own tone;
> And the tone vaporizes,
> Becomes a color image
> In the light—
> Light-gods-being.
>
> Vanished tone,
> In it resurrected tone
> Speaks out of it:
>
> You are
>
> Your own tone in the light of the world
> Tones radiating
> Radiate sounding.[80]

Finde dich im Lichte
mit der Seele Eigenton;
Und Ton zerstäubt
Wird Farbgebild
    Im Lichte —
Licht — Götter — Wesen.

Verschwundner Ton
In ihm wiedererstandener Ton
    Spricht aus ihm:
        Du bist
Eigenton im Wellenlicht
        Töne leuchtend
        leuchte tönend

Meditation by Rudolf Steiner. Ita Wegman manuscript
© Ita Wegman Archive, Arlesheim

The Principle of Hope

Adolescence, the time when one attains maturity in an earthly sense, has also always been the time of idealistic goals, of the foreshadowing of real possibilities and of concrete utopias in the sense of Ernst Bloch's "Principle of Hope." In his lectures on the anthropology of adolescence, Rudolf Steiner described the age-appropriate unfolding of the forces of love—not only in personal relationships but also far beyond, in the "experience of the whole of humanity" and in the "power of general human love."[81] He described the awakening of the "power of moral intuition" or of the "self-discovered good" at this time and explained:

> It was always to groups of human beings in association that the old intuitions were given. The new intuitions must be produced within each single, individual human soul. In other words, each single human being must be made the source of morality. This must be brought forth through intuitions out of the nothingness which humanity is facing.[82]

Young people are able to discover in themselves ideals that give life "direction and purpose out of itself," the "new intuitions." "Nothing is worse for later life than if these forces have not been there, have been missing, up to age twenty."[83]

One can and must ask oneself what the situation is today with regard to these youthful abilities—in view of a future that currently can neither be "planned" nor offers any perspectives at all, that seems completely open or even completely chaotic, and allows for almost no predictions—also because no one knows where and under what conditions he will be allowed to move about. In such a crisis, the youthful "love of action" mentioned by Steiner, "of that which is to become action, of that which is to become deed," is in a terrible situation. Nevertheless, despite—or precisely because of—generally poor prospects, the desire for a complete reorganization of civilization, for a new vision of society that leaves behind the old "history of separation" (Eisenstein) and sets out for other shores, was already shining in not a few young people's souls in the "Fridays for Future" movement. Charles Eisenstein speaks of a "society of participation" instead of domination, of living with the living Earth instead of destroying nature, of love instead of isolation. "The social climate, the political climate, the relational climate, the psychic climate, and the global climate are inseparable."[84] This insight currently lives in many sensitive young people, including the will to create a new society oriented in this way, where responsibility and empathy replace constriction, "authoritarianism," and militarization, where love of life and a science of the living is cultivated, not a science of death with its depletion of the life of the Earth and of human souls. *"You degrade nature, you tear it apart, there where patient Nature tolerates you, but it lives on"* (Hölderlin).[85]

Possibly, in such a mood, at some point the vision of "social threefolding" and with it the autonomous development of the three distinct spheres of society will reawaken—instead of the strong and centrally organized state or the all-powerful economy. The "Free Waldorf School" is a fragment that has emerged out of this new social conception,[86] a "fragment belonging to other contexts," as we might say, following Rilke. Rudolf Steiner counted preparing people for a "society of the future" among the challenges of the new school and spoke of the "great tasks of humanity" to be solved and of a "social deed of great style," the preparation of a "social spirit."[87] Steiner advocated the conception of a school free of the state, subject neither to the interests and dictates of the economy nor to those of the state, and an education that helped the children of today *"to become people of a new order of tomorrow"*[88] through a pedagogy of freedom and responsibility. In his lectures on the creation of a new society in the sense of social threefolding, he spoke of the necessary "love for the human social order"[89] and of the "objective public spirit,"[90] which are necessary for the development of a civil society of the future, but which are also made possible and promoted by this "new order." He also respected schools as places in which these abilities can be trained, thus also as real places of the future. It is a matter of preparing something "wholesome in the social structure of humankind"[91] in order to save the "living conditions of modern humankind" and to prevent "chaos and destruction," "dictatorships," "misery and annihilation."[92] Humankind is not at the end but "at the starting point of the greatest struggles, the spiritual struggles of the civilized world."[93] A completely new awareness of the value of human life on Earth is necessary, and also an awareness of "what is at stake today for the evolution of humankind."[94]

If we consider the overall dimension of the crisis in which humanity (and the biosphere) finds itself at the beginning of the third decade of the twenty-first century, Steiner's words do not seem antiquated but astonishingly topical, also with regard to schools and their tasks. Today's young people will not only have to persevere and endure in tomorrow's crisis-ridden world, but they can turn the situation around, on both a small and a large scale, provided they have the power of judgment and a "sense of truth," independence, creative imagination, creative ability, and the capacity for dialogue. The goal cannot be a return to "normality"—which even before Covid was highly pathological in many respects—but a fundamental change of that world which produces zoonoses, climate disruptions, socioeconomic, ethnic, and other authoritarian encroachments that are in themselves absurd, incredibly dangerous, and blatantly unjust. The motto of the future cannot be habituation to the unbearable, but rather the goal must be a new beginning from other forces and with another image of the human being, the Earth, and society. In the face of these enormous challenges, it is not acceptable for us in our school communities or as a society to fall out completely over the wearing or not-wearing of masks and to waste all our energies on what is really a side issue—however unpleasant or symptomatic, and thus significant, it may be; above all, we must not lose sight of what is actually at stake here. We must not allow ourselves to be distracted from the real issue, which is in need of change and which is spoken of far too seldom, even in schools, in my opinion.

It will and must always be left to young people to find their "moral intuitions" themselves, and it can by no means be their generational task to implement the visions of their predecessors that have not yet been realized, not even those of viable and meaningful concepts such as "social threefolding." Nevertheless, it seems obvious to me that young people must be given conceptual stimuli and encouragement, measures of a meaningful life and images of concrete utopias inside and outside of school, contoured images that young people can transform and shape in their own way, radically reject or independently reinvent. It seems to me to be of central importance that schools become places in which we seek to understand the complexities of reality—thus also the reality of the Covid crisis—but that they are also places which stimulate and challenge our creative imagination, including our creative imagination for coping with sociopolitical and ecological tasks and problems; that schools become places which look the difficult reality in the face and at the same time carry the breath of freedom, courage, hope, confidence, and tolerance—yes, the art and joy of living. Such schools belong to the civil society of the future and are urgently needed.

A desire for the "restoration of a shared world" currently lives in many young people, that much I can say from my own experience. As Charles Eisenstein wrote in March 2020:

> Yes, we can proceed as before down the path toward greater insulation, isolation, domination, and separation. We can normalize heightened levels of separation and control, believe that they are necessary to keep us safe, and accept a world in which we are afraid to be near each other. Or we can take advantage of this pause, this break in normal, to turn onto a path of reunion, of holism, of the restoring of lost connections, of the repair of community and the rejoining of the web of life.[95]

Addendum

Civil Courage

The Challenge of Independent Waldorf Schools

Author's presentation of a lecture on July 25, 2020, at the Rudolf Steiner Haus Stuttgart, within a colloquium organized by Dr. Armin Husemann, MD, on the pedagogical consequences of the Covid crisis.

It may seem strange, at the end of a colloquium on the educational consequences of the Covid crisis—including the problem of digital learning—to hear a presentation on the resilience and creative resistance of Waldorf schools in the Nazi era, especially since the historical situations and challenges then and now are completely different. Nevertheless: "History does not repeat, but it does instruct" (Timothy Snyder).

Personally, I would have liked to have presented the main elements of this lecture last year, in the context of the "Waldorf 100" centenary and the various events which marked the occasion, but interest in the topic of Nazi history was and is not very great in the Waldorf movement. Nevertheless, in 2019 I was able to publish my extensive monograph *Erzwungene Schließung: Die Ansprachen der Stuttgarter Lehrer nach dem Ende der Waldorfschule im deutschen Faschismus (1938)* [Forced closure: The speeches of Stuttgart teachers after the end of the Waldorf School under German fascism (1938)], which takes up and continues the research into National Socialism conducted by Norbert Deuchert, Uwe Werner, Wenzel Götte, Karen Priestman, and Volker Frielingsdorf.

The book appeared—completely unintentionally—on the day of the first Waldorf school's centenary, September 7, 2019. It examines the behavior of Waldorf schools in the Third Reich, and I still believe that this should have been addressed intensively and publicly last year from our side; we would not have then been so defenselessly exposed to the eternally recurring accusations of racism and anti-Semitism, and very many parents and teachers—and also high school students—would have learned something important about their "Free School" under a totalitarian, unfree government. They would have then known more about the very difficult situation in which the Waldorf school movement in Germany, with its nine schools, found itself in 1933, approximately fourteen years after its founding; and—contrary to all the distortions by today's critics—they would also have learned a lot about the resilience and the creative means of resistance that Waldorf schools were quite remarkably capable of between 1933 and 1941, until the closure of the last school in Dresden.

The topic seemed to me to be important in 2019 also because of the general political developments, the renewed strengthening of authoritarian right-wing nationalism and extremism, also in Germany—just think of the last AfD election results in Thuringia, the state of Weimar and Jena, but also of Buchenwald! This political development raised the question for me: How long will there be "Free Schools" in the future at all, *if* this tendency continues and spreads further, and *if* one wants to continue to use the term "Free" or "Independent Waldorf School" at all? It is a well-known fact that this freedom is not readily accepted in many respects.

~

The topic of National Socialism, however, was and remains unpopular, although it is so eminently important, especially for the future. Why is it so unpopular, you may ask? I think that a general *forgetfulness* or *disillusionment with history* plays a not insignificant role here, also within the anthroposophic movement or rather "scene"; looking back is only conditionally desired here. One longs, quite justifiably I think, for the present and the future, for what is needed today and tomorrow, and not for old stories, not for memories or glorification, of which one has heard often enough and which often helps so little when it comes to coping with our *present* tasks, with the people who are actually here today. As understandable as all this is, it is, on the other hand, problematic and even dangerous.

Without a historical and life-historical consciousness, human beings and society as a whole would wander around, repeating the old mistakes, missing their realizations, yes, their "'I'-becoming" within time and through time; that is what I, as a psychiatrist and psychotherapist, would like to consider at this point. One could quote Friedrich Schiller, this man of the future, who lived, forward-looking, with so much energy, with so much creative power, and at the same time with an eminent awareness of history. Or Rudolf Steiner or Novalis, or many others. I do not want to speak here of the fact that history, from an anthroposophic perspective, is also—if not primarily—a realm of destiny; what our predecessors did or did not do, also in the domain of Waldorf schools, concerns us, has to do with us, and is not mere "history."

However, the retrospective study and discussion of human behavior is not only relatively unpopular in Germany today but has been for more than seventy years. In this respect, Waldorf schools share Germany's social lot; concealment and repression of the recent past has been pervasive since 1949 at the latest. I think that at that time, in the first years after 1945, after their readmission, the Waldorf school communities, the teachers and the parents, essentially gathered all their forces over and above their differences in order to be able to reopen and lead the schools again. They invested all their forces in reconstruction and not in retrospection, reflection, and self-criticism. As I said, this was done in accordance with the general behavior in Germany, with the leading "paradigm," albeit in a special way—for it was not done in the spirit of the "economic miracle" but out of a sense of responsibility for an extremely important and demanding pedagogy. Moreover, I am of the opinion that shame played a not inconsiderable role in this and that it continued to have an effect for a very long time—indeed, right into our own time. Did the Waldorf schools have reason to be ashamed, you may ask, a special reason to be ashamed beyond the general reason in Germany?

Yes, I think that shame was indeed present for a time within our anthroposophic school movement, or at least within the community of teachers, and I will give you the following reasons, some reasons that seem at least plausible to me.

For one thing: Most of the approximately 160 Waldorf teachers were relatively surprised by and unprepared for the political situation in 1933 and in the years that followed—despite countless warnings from Rudolf Steiner and individual members of his staff about such a situation, including not least of all Ita Wegman, who saw through the political developments early on. At least some of the teaching staff apparently did not yet recognize the political situation in 1933, did not have the necessary awareness of the problem; some were politically naïve, preoccupied with their school and little else. They underestimated, as did very many Germans—indeed, as did the overwhelming majority of the German population—the danger of the new government under Hitler, relying on idealism, even the apparent idealism of the early Nazi period. After 1945, one could be ashamed of it; after 1945— and already in the last years of the National Socialist tyranny—everything was very clear, in the light of the Holocaust, the World War, and the political persecution. But then it was also definitely too late. Rudolf Steiner had expected something different, and timelier, from Waldorf teachers; he had worked tirelessly for a pronounced power of judgment toward sociopolitical processes—*contemporary* sociopolitical processes— and had given countless lectures and had written books on this subject. The "darkness of the lived moment" of which Ernst Bloch speaks, however, was and remained apparently impenetrable for most listeners.

What the situation in the faculty rooms of the Waldorf schools actually was around 1933, how the Nazi regime was assessed, we admittedly do not know in detail to this day; no minutes were recorded during meetings on the subject, for good reason. The Waldorf teachers, it seems to me, concentrated on maintaining their school, under the new circumstances, which for them—in contrast to the majority of Germans— became extraordinarily difficult already a few weeks after the National Socialist takeover; they were extremely busy and therefore possibly narrowed their horizons, improvising from day to day. We can understand that—we can perhaps understand it very well

today in particular, which I will come back to later—
but it was not sufficient, as became clear to them in
the end, shamefully clear.

I also think that many Waldorf school teachers were
ashamed after 1945 because they had been so intensely
fearful of state power in 1933 and in the following
years, of restrictions, visitations, and summonses that
began shortly after the National Socialists came to
power. The Anthroposophical Society was banned in
November 1935, after lengthy preparations by Himmler and Heydrich; card indexes of anthroposophists
by name existed, and extensive searches and seizures
took place, including many interrogations. Waldorf
teachers were afraid and the majority tended toward
an "almost Lutheran acceptance of state rule," as Wenzel Götte accurately put it. In the first years of Nazi
rule, they predominantly chose the path—if it was a
real "choice"—of fearful adaptation, of survival prag-
matism, and opportunism.

We can condemn this and very probably the teachers
themselves condemned it after 1945—or were ashamed
of it. But, what else should they have done? And what
would we have done in this situation? Of course, they
could have simply closed their "Free Waldorf Schools"
after January 30, 1933, and handed over all their students to the state schools, all these children and young
people, to the institutions of indoctrination planned by
Hitler, Goebbels, Baldur von Schirach, Bernhard Rust,
and others. But was that a real alternative? Would we

have done that? Will we close our schools in the future if—under completely different political circumstances—we find ourselves in situations in which actual Waldorf education, as an education for freedom and community, is no longer possible or no longer permitted?

The situation at that time was extremely delicate; we should never forget that fact in historical retrospect. The teachers, together with the parents and the sponsors of the schools, bore the responsibility for a special new pedagogy, which seemed vital to them and for the children entrusted to them. They therefore first took the path of preservation and acceptance and therefore accepted the *Gleichschaltung* (synchronization)* of 1933. In order to continue to exist, the Waldorf schools had to join the NSLB, the *Nationalsozialistischen Lehrerbund* [National Socialist Teachers' Association], which would never have occurred to them without absolute coercion. They could have refused, but as private schools, they would have been closed immediately, still in the first half of 1933, without exception. They therefore "chose" to join the NSLB and for this they first had to form an umbrella organization, which they had never had before and never needed, the *Reichsverband der Waldorfschulen* [Imperial Association of Waldorf Schools], which was soon renamed *Bund der Waldorfschulen* [Federation of Waldorf Schools]; this, and nothing else, is the

---

* The term *Gleichschaltung* (meaning "coordination" or "synchronization") refers to a process of Nazification designed to turn Germany into a single party state under Hitler and the Nazi Party.

antecedent of today's *Bund der Freien Waldorfschulen* [Association of Independent Waldorf Schools]—it was a necessary, forced association to adapt to the circumstances.

The teachers also had to do something else that I suspect they were later ashamed of: they had to start the school day with "Heil Hitler!" Starting in 1936, they had to take the so-called "loyalty oath" to Hitler. Also, as early as 1934, they had to separate themselves from all colleagues who had a Jewish or part-Jewish family background so that the Waldorf schools could continue to exist. They finally decided to do so—and in Stuttgart in 1934, Karl Schubert, Friedrich Hiebel, Ernst Lehrs, and Alexander Strakosch left the school. The Waldorf teachers cared for these highly esteemed and beloved colleagues, professionally, economically, and on a human level, which was by no means a matter of course at that time; they were far from inwardly distancing themselves from them or defaming them. Nevertheless, I think they were ashamed later on for accepting the forced dismissal of their colleagues, or rather their resignation (which the latter submitted in order to protect the school itself), even though they had no alternative other than closing the school.

They were also ashamed after 1945, I believe, of the numerous submissions that many of their representatives had made to ministries and other offices from 1933 onward in order to prove, at least rhetorically, the compatibility of Waldorf schools with the "new Germany." Some of these submissions were outright acts of self-denial and self-alienation; what they said about the meaning, goal, and origin of Waldorf education was in no way true but was often precisely the opposite of the truth, a fact the authors were well aware of. Nevertheless, they professed in their letters that their schools very much wanted to place themselves at the disposal of the "national uprising," that they had always been educating young people with "leadership qualities" in the sense of the German *Volksgeist*, etc. I will spare you the rest and refer you to the secondary literature mentioned earlier. With their written manifestos and their rhetoric of adaptation, the Waldorf school representatives convinced virtually no one in the ministries, at the party headquarters of the NSDAP, at the SS, the SD,* and in the Reich Security Main Office. As documents show, this lip service by anthroposophists was not taken seriously. Nevertheless, individual representatives of the "Bund" (Association) took this path.

Those involved were very probably also ashamed in 1945 of their temporary efforts to claim for the Waldorf school movement the young Nazi "martyr"

---

* The NSDAP (*Nationalsozialistische Deutsche Arbeiterpartei* [National Socialist German Workers' Party]) was a far-right political party in Germany, active between 1920 and 1945, that created and supported the ideology of Nazism. The SS (*Schutzstaffel* [Protection Squadron]) was the Nazi Party's elite paramilitary led by Heinrich Himmler. The SD (*Sicherheitsdienst* [Security Service]) was a subgroup of the SS. As the intelligence service of the SS, the SD was responsible for gathering intelligence about the Nazi Party's enemies, real and perceived.

Hans-Eberhard Maikowski, who had belonged to the SA** and had been shot on January 30, 1933. Those involved knew full well that he had only been at the Stuttgart Waldorf School for eleven months and— according to his tenth-grade report—had not been able to enter into the "spirit" of the school and had turned away and distanced himself.

They were also ashamed of the years of negotiations between the head of the Dresden Waldorf School, Elisabeth Klein, and leading representatives of the regime, including such prominent National Socialists and ideologues as Otto Ohlendorf and Alfred Baeumler. The teaching staff had essentially supported Elisabeth Klein's course of action for years, but after 1945 the majority no longer wanted anything to do with her as an alleged collaborator. Klein had tried not only to save her Dresden school from closure but to get it recognized as a "state experimental school," virtually as a "model school"; she had made an impression on her interlocutors and school inspectors through her manner and her pedagogical qualifications, including the qualities of the Dresden school, even though she was not, and never became, a National Socialist.

In the years after 1945, Waldorf teachers did not want to talk about Elisabeth Klein or her role, either internally or in public—just as they did not want to talk

---

** The SA (*Sturmabteilung* [Storm (or "Strike") Division]) was the Nazi Party's original paramilitary wing, effectively superseded by the SS in 1934, but continuing to exist until disbanded by the Allied Control Council in 1945.

about the Stuttgart School's temporary attempt to use the National Socialist portion of the parent body, which was very small but nevertheless present, to represent the school to the outside world. A parent like Leo Tölke, who had four children at the school and belonged to the SA, and a prominent anthroposophist and school supporter like the factory owner Hermann Mahle, took teachers to task for their critical statements against the regime. They convened Nazi parents' meetings and tried to enforce the National Socialist *Gleichschaltung* (synchronization) of the school board, with the ultimate aim of placing the school leadership into the hands of Nazi-affiliated parents and sponsors. The spiritual and social disintegration of the Stuttgart School was a real possibility in 1935, a "perishing from within," as the teacher Hermann von Baravalle accurately put it at the time. It was no longer possible to speak openly at the school about the problem. The system of denunciation had been established, and the Nazi representatives temporarily gained influence and power before they had to withdraw again, after a final objection by Emil Molt and a decisive statement by the teaching staff.

I enumerate these difficult points here only briefly; they can—and should—be read in detail. The reappraisal of these things, which, as I emphasized before, has been carried out by various anthroposophic authors, is important—and I have written about Elisabeth Klein, for example, and her relation to Baeumler and Ohlendorf in some detail in the book *Erzwungene Schließung*

[Forced closure], which was written in the context of larger Nazi studies by our Institute.

Finally, to come back to the motif of shame one last time, I would like to emphasize at this point for people who have not yet looked into it that the detailed historical reappraisal of the Nazi period and the behavior of Waldorf schools at that time began very late—to my knowledge, with Norbert Deuchert's first and detailed publications in the mid-1980s—and that this took place under pressure from outside, in the wake of the critical Nazi inquiries of that time, in the decade after the APO.* For a long time, the Anthroposophical Society and the Waldorf school movement were only marginally interested in this topic—very wrongly, in my opinion—and lagged behind, thus awakening the general suspicion of critics.

≈

Fair enough, you may say, or rather not so "fair," but why bring all of this up in the context of a colloquium on the educational consequences of the Covid crisis? Isn't the topic I have discussed completely out of place here? Many people today are more than a little upset if such topics are even mentioned in the current crisis

---

* The APO (*Außerparlamentarische Opposition* [Extra-parliamentary Opposition]) was a political protest movement in West Germany during the 1960s and early 1970s, often synonymous with the West German student movement. It formed in opposition to the "grand coalition" government in power and, amongst other things, criticized the suppression of the crimes of National Socialism.

or brought into any connection with it. True, they say, the Covid measures involve far-reaching restrictions on basic rights and freedoms, but we definitely do not live in a dictatorial system in Germany; instead, we are extremely happy about our free and democratic constitution, especially in these times—and they are absolutely right about that. They also point out that the present is definitely not about the exclusion and persecution of groups of people but about protection against viruses—that is, not about the destruction of life but quite the opposite, about the preservation of life.

I understand these views very well—they are easy to understand and are obvious, so to speak. However, I think, on the other hand, one must also accept that, especially at the present time, people remember specific phenomena of the past, and I was therefore very happy to accept an invitation to this colloquium. One cannot compare current events with the events of 1933 to 1945 or see them as one. But neither can one merely be indignant toward people who point out that in the wake of the Covid measures we experienced the second closure of Waldorf schools, and that after their partial reopening we are dealing with serious interventions in the curriculum, indeed in the whole school community—with interventions such as we have experienced only once before in German history, albeit under quite different circumstances. Nor, I think, can we close our eyes to the fact that since March 2020 we have had to contend with a considerable monopolization of public opinion, including scientific opinion. "What is frightening is the intolerance and radicalism with which the results of other researchers and third-party opinions are defamed and discredited, as if critical scientific discourse were suddenly obsolete," writes observer Christiane Haid. We are indeed witnessing a demotion and discrimination of dissenters, a defamation carried out, according to the concerned infectious disease epidemiologist Sucharit Bhakdi, with "remarkable determination," which in part continued in Waldorf schools after their reopening. "Every person shall have the right freely to express and disseminate his opinions in speech, writing, and pictures.... There shall be no censorship" (Basic Law [of the Federal Republic of Germany], Article 5*). Is that still true, given the many reports on the internet that have been deleted because they are undesirable and do not correspond to the mainstream narrative?

Furthermore, I believe one cannot overlook the fact that there are currently many cases of fearful conformity and "anticipatory obedience," to the point

---

* On December 10, 1948, the United Nations General Assembly met in Paris to sign a unique document, the Universal Declaration of Human Rights. Born of the terrible experiences of the Second World War, this statement of principles was to form the foundation upon which democratic societies could grow. Article 19 states: "Everyone has the right to freedom of opinion and expression; this right includes freedom to hold opinions without interference and to seek, receive and impart information and ideas through any media and regardless of frontiers." Freedom of expression and its twin, freedom of the press, are accordingly an inalienable right of all people. They are enshrined in Article 5 of the German Basic Law.

of self-censorship, also in the Waldorf school movement—and that school communities thus enter into a
tense situation, which contains within it the potential
for a complete rupture of the previous cohesion. One
can currently experience in many Waldorf schools how
little open dialogue about the current situation is possible, or how intensively it is avoided—incidentally also
with the students, who actually have an absolute right
to comprehensive, multifaceted information, reflection, and free determination of where they stand, especially at a "free school" in times of real crisis in society.
"Many conversations today are already over after an initial inquiry—the worldview of one appears too incompatible with that of the other," is how Gerald Häfner
describes the situation. Alienation and also mistrust
and mutual surveillance, which are systematically promoted by certain forces in the current crisis, has even
invaded some Waldorf schools.

Of course, it is possible to consider this brief sketch
of the situation as a dramatization; one can point to
important exceptions in individual schools and colleges,
or read the beautiful reports in the magazine *Erziehungskunst*, which have nothing to do with the subject; one can also be content with simply being glad that
some form of school is allowed again at all and that our
situation is so much better than that in São Paulo; and
one can count on the further "loosening" of restrictions
and "normalization"—and on the fact that everything
will soon pass and not come back again.

Finally, one can add that the school break during the "lockdown" was an intensive family time, a "deceleration," and recreation, in the house and in the garden, under blue, airplane-free skies, in free nature—but only for the privileged among us, the socially and economically privileged, of whom there are, however, many in Waldorf schools, unlike in the early days of the Waldorf Astoria cigarette factory and its working families, who lived in cramped apartments. The professional presentations of this symposium also speak quite clearly, in my opinion, against a purely positive, largely class-specific interpretation of the situation.

What also speaks against such an interpretation is the experience of children and adolescents, even of children and adolescents from privileged families, who, despite all family and digital support, most definitely experience the seriousness of the situation—the real rupture of their previous lives, friendships, and activities, the break in society. One could see, after its closure, how important the school was and is for the children and young people, how central is the friendship and social space, the community of the class; it was anything but an unexpected, happy vacation and family time for most of them, not even for children who were protected from the epidemic of fear.

As a trained child and adolescent psychiatrist and psychotherapist, I believe we tend to overlook the depth of the traumatic experience, beneath the seemingly wholesome surface, in a positively colored interpretation of the situation. One should not under-estimate today's children and young people—they were born into an age of extremes, of upheavals, and not into an "ideal world." They know more about it than we generally suspect. This is shown not least by the youth protests against the climate catastrophe, which in my opinion should also be taken much more seri-ously in Waldorf schools.

Finally, in my opinion, the view of the extremely serious economic, ecological, sociopolitical, and also biotechnological dimension of the crisis speaks against defaming people who point out the problems of the situation and of certain perspectives and are definitely *not* the "covidiots" and "Covid deniers" that they are made out to be by the media. Whoever even begins to survey the corresponding developments knows what concepts of biotechnological monitoring and complete control—and also of invasive "human technology" and "transhumanism"—have long since ceased to be mere possibilities.

> In China, one must already have an app on one's cell phone that permanently displays the owner's risk of infection in the colors red, yellow, or green. The authorities decide on the assignment without listening to the owner or allowing him to object. Those for whom the cell phone glows red are no longer allowed to use public transportation. They are also no longer allowed to enter public spaces or stores. They are prevented from doing so on the basis of an automated decision. And that's just

a first taste. We will have to deal with even more
far-reaching dangers and tendencies in the future.
(Gerald Häfner)

To disqualify as "conspiracy theorists" those who
have objectively familiarized themselves with these
clear dangers to humanity is completely absurd; here
it is simply a matter of a necessary knowledge of the
dangers of modern civilization, to which I would like
to return later.

No, we are certainly not experiencing a relapse into
the years around 1933, but nevertheless we are facing
an extremely serious situation, a global "narrowing of
politics" in the direction of technocracy, as Gerald Häfner writes. I therefore plead that we not simply silence
or condemn to silence those who have experienced
times of political totalitarianism—among them not a
few people in the former German Democratic Republic,
as I know from conversations with Waldorf teachers in
East Germany. One can also leave aside the emotion-
ally-loaded concept of totalitarianism; but the fact that
"total forces" tend to be effective in the rules of virolo-
gists and hygienists, that a total system in its complete
and tremendous one-sidedness is at work here is evident
to many people, even to those who consider the measures—from "social distancing" to masking—to be an
unavoidable evil. All specialized disciplines, when they
become all-powerful, tend toward "totality." If one were
to reorganize the whole of society, for example, according to the rules, priorities, and guidelines of insurance

agents or constitutional protectionists or geneticists, one would be surprised how different our everyday existence would become. We have already become accustomed to the fact that our world has long since been structured and organized according to the rules of the economy and industry; "total" forces are also at work in them, which take no account of anything else, as we are well aware, because only one goal counts and everything else becomes secondary or tertiary, "irrelevant," or "not relevant to the system." This is no different with virology—and it is exceedingly dangerous for society as a whole. Waldorf educators Florian Oswald and Claus-Peter Röh emphasize: "With the virus, the method of how to fight it was also immediately dictated. Suddenly a dogmatic, totalitarian approach exerts its influence and infects democratic systems."

~

This brings us back to the situation in schools. I believe that large parts of the Waldorf school movement in Germany, despite many differences, have also gained common insights in recent months, among which, after the joyful events of the "Waldorf 100," I would include the following three insights. I realize they are anything but new, but they nevertheless became clearer in the acute crisis:

1. The "Independent Waldorf Schools" are by no means "free" or "independent" but, like all schools, can be closed by the state at any time; moreover, they

are anything but "free" in their curriculum design. What is considered "system-relevant" and, for example, may or must be taught within a time frame determined by Covid regulations is decided by this "system" and not by the school, even if the latter views subjects such as art and religion as essential for child development and health, for salutogenesis and resilience. Whether we can truthfully call the Waldorf schools existing today "free" or "independent" needs to be fundamentally reconsidered—something Valentin Wember has been saying for years.

2. The principle of the teachers "collegial leadership" was not, or not sufficiently, effective in the time of crisis in many places, because either no more meetings took place at all or a common understanding among the teachers about the extent and the character of the crisis did not arise—and the difficult topic, with its tremendous power to generate social discord, was avoided in many places in order to preserve at least some social cohesion.

3. The so-called "school community" is an extremely fragile entity. Many parents and not a few high school students feel left out of this community in central questions of decision-making and future goals, especially in times of crisis—and the principle of internal parent representative bodies and committees can become a world of its own with its own specific dynamic that is not able to solve or replace the fundamental challenge

of a school *community*, which is part of the conception of the Waldorf school.

One can indignantly negate these critical points—and other painful aspects, including the very limited foundational anthroposophic work and substance in the schools—or one can contritely acknowledge them and melancholically regret them; one can furthermore blame them on the overstrained Waldorf schools and teacher colleges; however, none of these approaches will lead anywhere. Instead, it seems important to me to admit the facts as such and not to cover them up or pass them over. Crises always also hold opportunities, can lead to necessary changes, out of necessity. "*Show your wound*," said Joseph Beuys, whom we should not forget.

≈

Personally—and I would like to emphasize this at this point—in recent months I have grown to respect, and in some cases even to hold in high esteem, what the Waldorf schools accomplished from 1933 to 1941, and I have come to understand anew, and perhaps for the first time, how difficult it must have been to hold on to Anthroposophy, Waldorf education, and its humanistic view of the human being in the face of the overwhelming majority of opponents at that time, against the enormous pressure to conform, and in the face of rampant fears and repression. Today one underestimates the suggestive pull of the nationalistic, but also the "social-hygienic" thinking of that time, which in no way argued for the extermination but rather for the preservation and health of the "people's body," with severe "hereditary ailments" and eugenic perspectives—and was thereby considered scientific, as the "state of science." I understand the aspects of shame after 1945 that I have enumerated above and that are very likely not complete, but I still believe that one should look much more closely at the historical "wound" of the German Waldorf schools, if it is a "wound" at all. In fact, from today's perspective, the schools unfolded an astonishing degree of resilience and creative resistance, and a closer look reveals what gross oversimplification and actual slander it is to claim that Waldorf schools took the "path of least resistance with the simultaneous presence of anti-Semitism and German nationalism" from 1933 to 1941 (Ansgar Martins). There is no cause for anthroposophic arrogance and arrogant self-aggrandizement ("we were immune to National Socialism")—on the contrary. However, a few important points remain to be noted:

1. Not a single Waldorf school teacher, according to the findings of the historical studies available to date, was an avowed National Socialist. The Nazi-affiliated teacher Els Moll was dismissed in Stuttgart, and the "uprising" of the small but active National Socialist parents was overcome in Stuttgart. Nor did it stand a chance at any of the other Waldorf schools.

2. The internal protest from the ranks of Waldorf teachers against ingratiating and self-denying appeals to the authorities from individual school representatives was, as the documents show, already great in 1933 and gained intensity in the following years, including the protest against the actions of Elisabeth Klein. Discussions about how far to go in outward conformity and to what extent to even begin to accept the separation of Waldorf education from Anthroposophy (which was considered an "enemy of the state" or "subversive of the state") were vehement. The vast majority of Waldorf teachers unequivocally rejected the idea of a state "experimental school" as pursued by Klein; the historical documents show this unequivocally (see my monograph *Erzwungene Schließung* [Forced closure]).

3. It was not only the Jewish members of the teaching staff who belonged fully to the Waldorf school community—until their forced resignation by the state—but also Jewish school children, who often received special care and protection. "The school was the only safe place for me," reads the recollection of a former Waldorf teacher from a Jewish family, which I quote from my aforementioned book. It is known of Karl Ege, the Stuttgart teacher, that he always very consciously and emphatically gave the main roles in the plays of his class to a Jewish, socially marginalized child. About her teacher Clara Düberg, a former Berlin Waldorf pupil wrote, "One day Fräulein Düberg, the only older teacher, stood before us. Eerily, she let loose a rage, the

tall slender figure with the waving white bush of hair—
an unforgettable image: 'Who said to one of my boys
"you old Jew"?' She clenched her fists, she screamed,
ran menacingly back and forth. Our blood froze in our
veins. How often I had to say to myself: 'What would
have been prevented in Germany if all the teachers had
shouted like that?'" Anna-Sophia Bäuerle also reported
that on class trips with overnight stays, the whole class
slept on straw beds in farms, "since Jewish students
were no longer accepted in the youth hostels." Nor were
all Waldorf teachers in 1933 and in the years that followed overstrained in their assessment of the political
situation; on the contrary, it is known how critical various prominent teachers were of the regime, including
Eugen Kolisko and Hans Rutz.

4. The Waldorf schools submitted individual opportu-
nistic and ingratiating petitions to state authorities, and
they had to make not inconsiderable concessions. However, their pedagogical concessions to the authorities
apparently ended at the gate of the school building—for
they continued their actual work there with the children and young people in an astonishingly uncompro-
mising manner. I wrote about this in my study on the
"forced closure":

> Wenzel M. Götte, who, following Norbert Deuc-
> hert, further evaluated the critical state audit
> reports on the Waldorf schools, came to the
> conclusion that according to the reports, the
> schools—including Elisabeth Klein's school in

Dresden—showed no willingness whatsoever to "change anything *substantially*" during the Nazi years. Although the obvious course of action would have been to meet corresponding expectations at least during the visit of the inspectors from the state and the party, this clearly did not happen within the lessons. Thus, the eleventh-grade history lesson in the Stuttgart Waldorf School was severely reprimanded by the inspector at the end of April 1935; among other things, he wrote, commenting: "The word *race* does not occur at all in the whole lesson." Also, in the Hamburg-Wandsbek Waldorf School in January 1937 "there was no sign of any attention to the ministerial regulations concerning the cultivation of German prehistory by evaluating the results of racial studies...." A "complete lack of any knowledge" of "early Germanic history" was recorded by the NSLB evaluator on this occasion; even of Frederick the Great and Bismarck as "heroes" of the German "spirit" in modern history, nothing had been heard.

As School Inspector Klussmann had already remarked in Hanover in February 1935, the Waldorf schools' cultural history lessons continued to take their unchanged course in the "new Germany"—and in their international and world-historical orientation, according to the inspector, the lessons went "far beyond the tasks of a *German* school." "The *Germanization* of the contents was missing, the subject of *race* was bypassed, history lessons still began with Eastern cultures in the fifth grade, even in local history an ideological penetration of the subject matter was dispensed with" (Götte). Steiner's guidelines, on which the curriculum was based, were and remained— despite all the petitions of the schools since 1933 and the intensive negotiations of individual school representatives—"foreign to those of the People's State and thus to those of a consciously German education." School Inspector Klussmann also had to note angrily that "the revised curricula in the state schools, the new textbooks, the banning of older ones" had "no effect" on the Waldorf schools because they had never used textbooks. This was also criticized by the Stuttgart School Council at the end of April 1935:

"The school has not found any reason since 1933 to apply for any new books, especially German reading or history books." Furthermore, the Stuttgart School Council did not find the English lessons of the teacher Erika von Baravalle "German" enough ("Unfortunately, already this first lesson shows that the lessons are not based on German feelings and German cultural heritage, but are fully rooted in the ideas of English-American school methods..."), and they were offended by the 'unmanly' eurythmy, which was not very committed to the spirit of soldiery—and by many other things. ("That one...expects German boys of seventeen or eighteen to imitate such dancing-like, soft movements, is something downright unnatural.")

The schools did not meet the "political pedagogy" of the Nazi regime, not only in the lessons but also in their atmosphere, which caused astonishment and indignation among the inspectors: "I ask myself how it is possible that a school in Germany can still be so far removed from the great events of our day and not have taken a step forward. Not a single drawing, not a single song, not a single poem, nothing revealed anything about what is going on in Germany today," remarked Marie Riemar, the *Gau** advisor for Education in the Nazi Teachers' Association, after her inspection of the Wandsbek Waldorf School on March 6, 1937. The morning lessons—also on the day of the audit—still began with a verse by Rudolf Steiner. Even in the large Stuttgart School, "appealing decorations with German pictures" were still missing in the classrooms, and the teachers' room still had "no picture of the Führer." In Hamburg-Wandsbek, it was indeed to be found in the teachers' room, but—like everything else—the school still did not meet expectations: "In none of the classrooms visited did a picture of the Führer hang, but in each one a picture of Rudolf Steiner and a Madonna. No classroom was decorated with a picture of a German landscape or a German hero. The picture of the Führer was only relatively small compared to the large picture of Rudolf Steiner in the teachers' room and also relatively small in the main entrance of the school." The NSLB reporter, who had accompanied School Inspector Thies in January 1937 during the inspection of the school in Wandsbek, continued: "In drawings, written notes, musical

* The *Gaue* (singular: *Gau*) were the main administrative divisions of Nazi Germany from 1934 to 1945.

and declamatory performances, anthroposophic ideas were quite conspicuously reflected, an indulgence in sweet and soft moods, a glorification of mere humanity and humankind. A battle song of our time was not heard. An elaboration of German traits was not recognized." "The method of education of the Stuttgart Waldorf School must be called international even today. Completely isolated, the Waldorf School stands in the face of the pulsating life of the *Volksgemeinschaft* [people's community]" a Stuttgart report said months later. Furthermore, the absence of an authoritative, controlling, and determining school leader in the sense of the "Führer principle" was criticized in Waldorf schools—which had, in fact, only formally adopted such a leadership principle. The treatment of the pupils was also considered too friendly: "The teacher takes all possible consideration of the pupils. They are hardly ever touched harshly, no strict discipline forces them to think for themselves," stated Ministerial Advisor Thies after visiting the Berlin Waldorf School in November 1934.

All in all, Thies' NSLB companion in Wandsbek, School Inspector Viernow, received the shocking impression in January 1937 that the Waldorf School had "remained untouched by the National Socialist spirit." The municipal official responsible in Stuttgart in February 1938 also saw "overwhelming evidence" for the necessary closure of the school. ("I am in agreement with the Württemberg Minister of Culture and all party and state authorities.")

Internally, the Waldorf schools were also extremely creative, independent, and resistant when it came to dealing with conditions that could not be radically resisted without risking premature closure (such as the Hitler salute before classes began, the raising of flags at the beginning of the week, the singing of the Germany and Horst Wessel* song, etc.). Lola Jaerschky from the Berlin Waldorf School described all the pros and cons discussed in the long conference sessions after each new decree. ("What happened in the case of rejection? How was it to be absorbed, to balance what was demanded?")

Finally, they endured the unpopular requirements and attempted to transform them internally: "One had to participate in the prescribed marches with the older students. One had to raise the flag in the presence of the whole school at the beginning and end of the school year. One had to listen to the radio broadcasts of certain speeches and take part in the prescribed celebrations. One had to conceal one's true opinion and be quick-witted in camouflaging remarks. One suffered from it, but one took it upon oneself, because there was no other way if one wanted to exist.... After all, it was not irrelevant how one did the inevitable. One could do it with embarrassment, briskly, or with verbalized gallows humor. One

---

*   Horst Wessel Song, also known by its opening words "Die Fahne hoch" [Raise the flag high], was the anthem of the Nazi Party (NSDAP) from 1930 to 1945. From 1933 to 1945, the Nazis made it the co-national anthem of Germany, along with the first stanza of the "Deutschlandlied" [Song of Germany].

could reinterpret words and symbols and hide
one's own meaning in them. But one could also
admit the whole untruthfulness and experience
the evil, the father of all deception, as a powerful opponent. When the Hitler salute was introduced, before and after every lesson—I mean
every lesson, including eurythmy and religion lessons—one raised one's arm in the consciousness
memento mori, the downfall is imminent."

Many of the pupils perceived the non-identi-
fication of their teachers with the corresponding
requirements; the way in which they "fulfilled"
them spoke for itself, without giving National
Socialist-minded parents objective grounds for
complaint and intervention. Every lesson had
to be started with "Heil Hitler" in a tight pos-
ture. Miss Siebert, for example, did this with a
very quick *"GoodmorningheilHitlersitdown,"*
wrote Johannes Kühne in a memoir of his Berlin
Waldorf School days.

Uwe Werner, who collected many reports
about corresponding behavior and who spoke
and corresponded with many people who had
been Waldorf students in the years 1933 to
1941, writes, "*The Song of Germany* was played
in Stuttgart as Joseph Haydn's *Kaiserquartett*
(Emperor Quartet)—which contains the original
music of the *Song*—with all its movements. For
this, one did not need to stand and raise one's
arm. Then they performed Schiller's *Tell*, a fight
for freedom against the occupying forces. A Jewish pupil played Tell's boy, who with the apple on
his head told his father to pull the trigger—he

was not afraid! In racial studies, Ernst Blümel covered Slavs, Eskimos, and specifically a Dinaric race found in Upper Austria and Bavaria, but not the Jewish race. When the Hitler salute had to be introduced, one student refused to raise her arm. Ernst Uehli, the Swiss teacher, let her do so for a few days, then he took her aside and said, meaningfully, 'As a Swiss citizen, I feel as badly about this as you do. However, the school is now so vulnerable that its chances of continuing to exist decrease if it comes out that someone at our school will not raise their arm. So, just raise your arm and think your piece!'"

Apart from this reminiscence of a special "racial studies" lesson by Ernst Blümel, not much has come to light about such a lesson at Waldorf schools. "Although the Waldorf schools, like the rest of the schools, were expected to teach *racial studies*, there is no evidence to suggest that they complied," wrote Karen Priestman after extensive source study. Lili Kolisko pointed out that her husband, Eugen Kolisko, resigned as school physician and teacher in Stuttgart in November 1934 partly because he felt he was being forced to include aspects of heredity and racial studies in his high school classes. ("Certain things had to be taught to the children with regard to heredity and also racial studies, especially in the upper classes and in the classes held in preparation for final exams. Dr. Kolisko could not reconcile this with his conscience as a Waldorf teacher.") Ernst Blümel, however, apparently subsequently solved the problem in his own way. Eugen Kolisko left the school in 1934 also for other reasons, not least as a result of the severe criticism he had received through his work for Ita Wegman, Elisabeth Vreede, and the "Free Working Communities" in the Anthroposophical Society.

On the subject of "racial studies" and a school booklet on it in the Hanover Waldorf School, the relevant literature states, "The inspector and head of training at the National Socialist Women's League around the district of Hanover City, Dr. Erna Sturm, reported that in a school booklet on racial studies, which also had to be introduced in Waldorf schools, she found no remarks on Judaism, on the meaning of racial care, on emergency population policy measures, but a sentence which seemed to her to be typical for the lessons: 'Bodily and mental characteristics are inherited, but the essence of the human being, his spirituality, belongs only to the individual.' The Nazi headmistress reacted with annoyance: 'The children are to be educated [in the Waldorf School] to become pan-Europeans and world republicans and for the international state.'"

It should also be noted that, according to the available reports, even after 1938 in Dresden, neither the school atmosphere nor the teaching changed, and this remained the case even when there were negative assessments by the school authorities and the NSLB. Despite her personal closeness to Baeumler,* Elisabeth Klein was

---

*   Alfred Baeumler (Nov. 19, 1887–Mar. 19, 1968) was an Austrian-born German philosopher, pedagogue, and prominent Nazi ideologue.

clearly not prepared to abandon the school's principles of autonomy. Baeumler's demands for a
complete reorganization of the curriculum—not
only in the subject of history—and for teaching
free of all "ties to Rudolf Steiner's worldview"
and only with teachers "who were able to commit
themselves wholeheartedly to National Socialism's historical view" were consistently under-
mined by Klein in Dresden and never became
reality; after the beginning of World War II, the
overburdened local authorities were busy with
other things, had no concrete concepts, and also
encountered internal resistance from Klein and
her faculty. Elisabeth Klein also kept the school
management in her hands and resisted any external takeover. The Dresden student memoirs of the
years 1938 to 1941 speak of intense experiences,
especially of an artistic nature, of the reality of
the inner school community and—at least among
individuals—of an awareness of the political situation. One could tell from student essays, which—
according to the teachers' announcements—were
to be sent "to Berlin," how they were to be written, and the hoisting and taking down of the flag
by the teachers was, according to the former student Johannes Lenz, always carried out in such
a way that there was no doubt about opposition to the regime. "At the Steiner School there
was hardly any talk about politics," Bernt von
Helmont wrote about his Berlin school days, yet
many students were obviously aware of the situation. Johannes Lenz even claimed, "Whoever had
gone through school like we did at the Dresden

School was protected from ideology in the Third Reich. We could not fall for the National Socialist ideology and went through the years until 1945 without any ideological blunders."

5. Nor should the behavior of the Waldorf schools during the Nazi era be overlooked in a historical assessment, in light of the fact that most Waldorf schools eventually closed their doors after years of compromise because they could no longer maintain the inner identity of their institution under the given conditions—and, after intensive discussion of the situation in the teachers' colleges, were not prepared to make further concessions (such as taking the now required "oath of allegiance" to Hitler). Franz Brumberg, who was the de facto head of the school in Hamburg-Altona, said in his address to the parents on April 6, 1936:

From its internal structure, the National Socialist state must lay claim to totality—that is, according to the views of the state, there must be no educational institutions that are not under the leadership of the state and its responsibility. Now, however, institutions like our school are based on the principle of freedom in teaching and for this reason have become impossible.

The teachers of the Berlin School voted a year later for the "voluntary" self-closing of *all* remaining Waldorf schools "in order to remain true to Rudolf Steiner's work," as they wrote to their Stuttgart colleagues on August 26, 1937. When the Hanover School closed and only agreed to prepare the existing pupils for the transition to state schools through "retraining courses," it withdrew its previous school name and wrote to the Ministry:

> We see ourselves compelled to prepare the pupils for retraining in state institutions and thus to have to introduce working principles that contradict the requirements of a healthy education in the sense of Rudolf Steiner's pedagogy. The teaching staff of the Hanover Waldorf School considers it its duty not to burden Rudolf Steiner's name and work with the compromises this would necessitate. It has therefore decided that, as of today, the name Freie Waldorfschule [Free Waldorf School], a name that carries with it a great honor and an obligation, will be discontinued. We note that the sole responsibility for the destruction of this German cultural asset lies with the responsible authorities.

6. It later became known that individual Waldorf teachers continued to work with children and young people after the closure of their school, either in secret or semi-secretly. For example, three Berlin Waldorf teachers taught numerous "certified children"—who according to their "certification" needed special support—and far exceeded the maximum number of five children approved for this purpose; they also worked together with the children's parents on Rudolf Steiner's basic educational courses and designed a course for Jewish children in preparation for emigration to Palestine. The teachers who resisted in this way worked until their arrest in June 1941.

7. I would also evaluate as acts of resilience and creative resistance the last plays performed in the Stuttgart Waldorf School, in the months before closure, including Schiller's *Maid of Orleans* and Shakespeare's *Julius Caesar* (with their thematic leitmotifs of opposition and tyrannicide)—as well as the addresses of the Stuttgart teachers to their students after the school's closure in March 1938, all of which are included in my 2019 book *Erzwungene Schließung* [Forced closure]. In these addresses, the teachers' deep, unbroken, and undiminished respect for the essence of the Waldorf School becomes clear, for the "spirit of the school" and the essence of the children, for the educational task to which they felt committed—and not the guidelines and goals of the state. With their words, they gave the children and young people a great deal to sustain themselves inwardly in the near future in unfamiliar surroundings—and were inspired by the hope for the new beginning of the school after the end of the Nazi era.

One teacher's address spoke of reforging the "Grail Sword" in silence (Erich Gabert), and another of the necessity of continuing to carry the true image of the human being within oneself (Karl Ege). The school doctor, Gisbert Husemann, spoke of the "wand of Mercury" in the heart of each individual student, describing the force of truth as uprightness with love winding around it. Karl Schubert, in his memorial address for Rudolf Steiner, emphasized the "secret of being an undeceived human being" in the midst of a time of tremendous "seductions" and deceptions. It is, I think, very important to reread these speeches more than eight decades later. They give a sense of the inner strength of the school at the moment of its dissolution.

The Stuttgart students, all of whom attended the ceremony marking the closing of the school, never forgot it. Two of them, Friedhold Hahn and Johanna Maria Maier-Smits, then went to Berlin with a letter of protest from their class, wanting to talk to all the responsible politicians and dissuade them from their decision. Their teachers were against this dangerous plan, but Friedhold Hahn and Johanna Maria Maier-Smits could not be dissuaded from it. As their report shows, they really did go to individual ministries and at least got into the antechamber of those responsible, where they delivered their letter. They also reached Alfred Baeumler, the leading professor of political pedagogy—the only high National Socialist who had demonstrably studied Rudolf Steiner's work intensively. Baeumler had visited the Dresden Waldorf School with a commission and had written several expert reports on Anthroposophy and its applications; he also carried on a conversation with these two young people in his private apartment. He was impressed by them up to a certain point, by their school, by the work they had brought with them, which concerned the core of Anthroposophy and the core of National Socialism respectively, opposites that Baeumler—rightly—considered completely incompatible. At the end of the hour-long conversation, he finally asked Friedhold Hahn and Johanna Maria Maier-Smits if they would be willing, "without thinking, judging, or considering," to carry out an order for their Führer out of love and trust for Adolf Hitler. Johanna Maria Maier-Smit's report, written immediately after the trip, tells their short answer and Baeumler's reaction:

"No, we can't." He suddenly slammed the desk. "And that's why your school has to be closed!"

So ended the Berlin query and so ended the Stuttgart Waldorf School.

8. The Stuttgart Waldorf teacher Hans Rutz—whose teaching permit had already been withdrawn by the Württemberg Ministry of Education in 1937 (allegedly because of his Jewish "blood ties" but very likely as a result of a denunciation; among other things, he had opposed at his parents' evenings against the children's entry to the "Hitler Youth" and the "League of German Girls")—wrote the following lines from Goethe to his pupil Christhilde Blume's in her school yearbook on July 11, 1938:

> Cowardly thoughts,
> Nervous wavering,
> Meek trembling,
> Fearful lamentation
> Will not turn misery away,
> Will not set you free.
>
> Gathering all forces
> To keep you safe,

To never give way,
To show your strength—
This summons the arms
Of the gods.

I published these verses last year in Hans Rutz's handwriting in my book about the closing of the Waldorf School—it is worth taking a closer look. They are from Goethe's singspiel *Lila* and also played a role for Sophie Scholl and her friends—indeed, they were well known and considered important in German resistance circles.

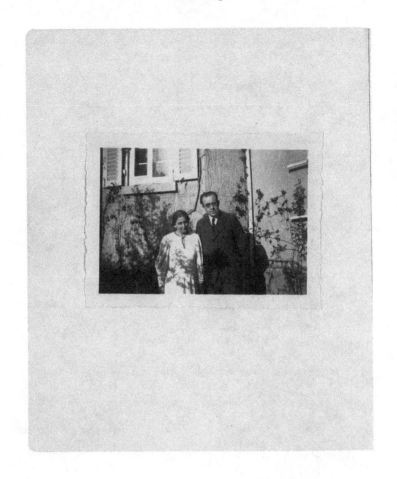

*Photograph of the teacher Hans Rutz and his entry in
the memorial book of the student Christhilde Blume
(© Archiv Waldorf School Stuttgart Uhlandshöhe)*

Feiger Gedanken
Bängliches Schwanken,
Weibisches Zagen,
Ängstliches Klagen
Wendet kein Elend
Macht dich nicht frei.

Allen Gewalten
Zum Trutz sich erhalten,
Nimmer sich beugen,
Kräftig sich zeigen,
Rufet die Arme
Der Götter herbei. (Goethe)

Der lieben Gottfried mit herzlichen
Wünschen!

Stuttgart, den 11ten Juli 1938.
Herta Ruth.

Entry ticket to the closing ceremony, March 31, 1938
© Archive of the Stuttgart Waldorf School Uhlandshöhe

With an abrupt leap into the present, into our present tasks and challenges, into the "acuteness of the present" (Paul Celan), we can ask ourselves whether we, too, must at some point begin to create books commemorating the Waldorf School. I have recently spoken with old Waldorf teachers who doubt whether the Waldorf school as such will survive the "Covid crisis"—because the prescribed measures strike at the heart of this special pedagogy and prevent it to a very considerable extent. In 1936, eighty-four years ago, the Stuttgart Waldorf teacher Ernst Uehli wrote:

> We can try to keep the Waldorf schools in Germany as long and only as long as the schools do not endanger the germinal power of the idea. If the compromises go so far and the school organisms

are so crippled internally and externally that the germinating power of the idea is endangered by their existence, then we must close.

No one, neither teachers nor the parents, wants to "close" a Waldorf School at the present time, but the "germinating power of the idea" is seen as threatened by many alert contemporaries. The Waldorf School is definitely not an institution for online learning; it works in a thoroughly radical way in terms of the human relationship; it relies on the principle of "I and Thou," in the language of Martin Buber, on the intensity of the encounter with individual students, with the community of the classroom, and the school as a vital whole; Waldorf education is based on closeness and not on distance. It works with art and creativity, with trust and confidence in life. It stands for a new way of thinking and for a new social spirit, also in dealing with science and technology, for a new health and vitality. It may be that the Covid measures will be completely lifted again and everything will continue as before, which is what many people hope for. But what is, in my opinion, much more likely is that the systems of security and control, "protection" and isolation, sterilization and "public hygiene," vaccination and behavioral standardization, digitalization and "distance learning" will remain to a considerable extent, at least latently as a possibility; they were not invented in the current Covid crisis but have been long in the making and follow corresponding aims and visions of society, which we can learn by looking, for example, at the Chinese state structure—in its technological infrastructure, its social norms of behavior, its economic efficiency, its maximum digitalization and control. All these forces and aspirations exist without any doubt, and they can generate a world in which real Waldorf education, its image of the human being, and its liberal life and social practice can no longer exist—can no longer exist and should no longer exist (well, perhaps a Waldorf education diluted beyond recognition, with some lessons on cultural epochs and individual musical instruments, movement art at a distance and online if necessary).

To completely ignore such a perspective or to indignantly oppose it seems to me incredibly naïve in view of the global situation and the social as well as technological developments of our time, including the biotechnological developments and visions of the future. I believe that *no* high school student of this clever and awake generation who has really looked around in the mentioned areas of concern would share such a naïve hope. It is extremely easy, with many decades of hindsight, to accuse people in 1933 of political cluelessness and ignorance, lack of judgment and perspective. But who among us today overlooks the context of what is coming? And who has the strength to stand against the current—especially when the "current" argues primarily or exclusively with medical-social perspectives, with the motives of "health" and the "protection of life," especially of those at risk, with aspirations that are shared by all of us—if not in this form.

≈

"Freedom *is* not but is always to be fought for," wrote Wenzel Götte in his excellent study on the question of the autonomy of the "Free Waldorf Schools," and the full truth of this sentence is shown by our present situation. At the beginning of June this year, the Waldorf school movement in Italy spoke out with a firm, socially engaged letter from its president, Claudia Gasparini, which went to a large number of government administrations. They, the Association of Italian Waldorf Schools and its president, are obviously not afraid of restrictions and defamation, and did this in the awareness that Rudolf Steiner also spoke out publicly during the founding period of the school and made himself very unpopular, although not with everyone. One also finds new friends, representatives of a free civil society, awake contemporaries, and allies against the general pressure to conform and adapt—this is also demonstrated by present experiences.

But how does one achieve access to the forces of creative resistance in difficult situations? How does one gain individual judgment in complex situations that do not permit simple answers, and how does one achieve real will and optimism for the future, beyond fearful conformity? I am convinced that it was Anthroposophy itself and the inner relationship with Rudolf Steiner, in his independent and extremely courageous approach, that decisively strengthened the Waldorf teachers after 1933 and helped them—indeed, all the school communities—to continue, even if they found themselves in an altogether powerless position after the National Socialists came to power. In the autumn of 1920, now one hundred years ago, Rudolf Steiner had once again emphasized in Dornach that in the near future the Waldorf school must develop the courage to pursue a real detachment from the state, in a new, tripartite form of society in which the spiritual-cultural life (to which all educational institutions belong) would work independently of the economic and the political-legal spheres—otherwise the whole Waldorf school movement would be "for the birds" (Oct. 12, 1920).

A few weeks earlier, Steiner had emphatically asserted in a Stuttgart teachers' conference that he was interested in a resolute representation of the concept of an autonomous school, but not in a "bow and scrape" before what was an "abomination" to Waldorf education (September 22, 1920). What came after 1933 was—in the first period of fearful adaptation and subordination—a clear "bowing and scraping" before "what was an abomination to us," before the colleges of teachers thought of something different and better. Today, too, Waldorf schools—even if under completely different political conditions and circumstances—find themselves in a situation that, as the contributions to this colloquium have demonstrated, is an "abomination" to real Waldorf education. Do we end at the "bowing and scraping" before the wave of digitalization and online education, before 5G and the so-called "requirements" of a technically defined modernity? And do we end at the "social distancing," the Plexiglas panes as protection for the isolated individual, at the measuring of classrooms and school-yards, the masked faces, the ever more divided groups, the actual end of the school community as a whole— and the compliance and implementation of countless administrative regulations that require all our energy and time and increasingly take the place of the former child studies, the place of real attention and humanistic pedagogy? What a situation for the teaching staff, and for the students and parents!

One can take the view that Waldorf schools currently have no choice but to hope that all this will not come about—at least not too quickly or too severely—and that much will continue to "loosen up" and "normalize"; one can even claim that everything in our Waldorf schools is going very well and—in view of the difficult circumstances—is basically "optimal" and that our schools should continue not to cause any offence and not to attract attention, not to develop any independent positions and so prevent any critical reporting about schools or Waldorf associations. If things ever turn out differently, however, one should not be surprised if in later times one is asked how one could have followed the majority opinions of the day and the compulsions to conform without resistance or reflection, how one could have been so faithful to individual scientific paradigms, and how, under the pressure of a "medicalized society" (Ivan Illich), one completely put aside all other considerations of the wellbeing of children and adolescents, of their social and developmental space, and even sacrificed the appropriate qualities instantaneously and largely without opposition. The question of whether there is still a need for Waldorf schools at all may also be asked in the future—for, as is well known, their foundation and expansion was only possible because Rudolf Steiner and his coworkers took a non-conformist, independent, and innovative path, in educational, scientific, and medical terms, a path that pursued values other than those already considered at the time to be the only ones that were "systemically relevant," and because Rudolf Steiner and his coworkers stood by these other values, and also publicly stood up for them in a proactive way (and naturally attracted much criticism).

Of course, it cannot be a matter of simply rejecting the ordinances today. Nevertheless, in the future we will very likely have to ask ourselves whether the adaptation and conformity, the docility and in some instances also the anticipatory obedience, in fear and trepidation, was really the right and *only* way in view of our pedagogical task.

But—you may ask—what then should and could Waldorf schools do today? Without claiming to have the right answers ready, four points seem urgent to me personally at the moment, as lessons from history and from reflection on the status quo.

First: A teacher at the Berlin Waldorf School, Herbert Schiele, wrote to Stuttgart in June 1936 that the task for the Waldorf school movement was to grasp the "spiritual character of the overall situation." This seems to me to be urgent also today—that we do everything possible to understand the "spiritual character of the overall situation" more deeply, instead of avoiding, as is currently done in many schools, any internal discussion of the Covid situation because such a discussion might increase the social tension of the school communities or the cracks between the different views. In fact, I think that we are most likely to find our way out of the polarity of viral panic—longing for total security (in a circumscribed area) and adaptation *versus* downplaying, fundamental opposition, and denial—through greater knowledge and by raising the level of reflection. One actually needs to know much more about virology and immunology than is reported in the plain and expedient media reports in order to be able to assess the situation more accurately—the efficiency, appropriateness, and problematic nature of some of the measures taken, including the testing procedures.

Thomas Hardtmuth, among others, has shown this impressively with his book *Corona und die Überwindung der Getrenntheit* [Covid and the overcoming of separateness], which he recently published with Christoph Hueck, Charles Eisenstein, and Andreas Neider.* I would see this as necessary reading for every Waldorf school community—that is, for *all* teachers and parents—in order to finally bring the internal school discussions to another level appropriate to a Waldorf school. If one reads the excellent essays by Hardtmuth, Hueck, and Eisenstein in this volume, one understands much more about the vaccination problem and the sociopsychological dynamics in which we currently find ourselves, of "ID 2020" and the ideology of control, of isolationism and social autism (in the sense of Reinhard Lempp's terminology).

As the leaders of the Pedagogical Section at the Goetheanum, Claus-Peter Röh and Florian Osswald, put it, "What the world is currently experiencing on a large scale is the installation of a control mechanism." Even if teachers and parents have never before dealt with these explosive fields of contemporary civilization—with trends and directions that existed long before Covid—after reading this slim book, they will understand more about the present age and the world in which we live and for which we must prepare our children and young people; they will then also understand more about the threat to free society posed by that "pathological mistrust of all against all," that

---

*   Not available in English; see, instead, Thomas Hardtmuth, *What Covid-19 Can Teach Us: Meeting the Virus with Fear or Informed Common Sense?*, trans. B. Jarman (Wynstones, 2021); also, Charles Eisenstein, *The Coronation: Essays from the Covid Moment* (Chelsea Green, 2022).

"xenophobia" as the "spiritual epidemic of the twentieth century," about which Stefan Zweig wrote long ago.
Furthermore, through Charles Eisenstein's presentation,
it becomes, I think, very clear that the present "war"
against the virus, as a "fight" against a defined enemy,
with its concentrated, maximal media-sharpened "call
for weapons," for subjugation, security, and maximum
control, follows a "logic of war," a highly problematic
pattern of conflict that we know extraordinarily well
from the—ultimately failed—political-military cam-
paigns of the last decades—from the fight against the
Taliban in Afghanistan, from the fight against the "axis
of evil," against Muammar Gaddafi or Saddam Hus-
sein. It was always about saving our supposedly exis-
tentially endangered "security" from a circumscribed
enemy, a one-dimensional rescue that was presented by
the governments involved with maximum media support as completely unavoidable, and it produced terrible
destruction—in the economic, social, ecological, and
political spheres. As Gerald Häfner writes:

> The reaction patterns [in the "war" against the
> virus] are the same everywhere; there are certainly
> nuances that tell us a lot about the mindset and
> character of certain politicians, about the culture
> of a country, and about the maturity of a soci-
> ety, but the aggressively combative mindset pre-
> dominates. This reveals a pattern of thought and
> reaction that cultivates a hostile relationship to
> the world, a combative approach, and defensive
> or domineering behavior. Everything that cannot

be integrated into the framework of the familiar worldview is blotted out or destroyed. What happens is the opposite of what could or should be done in an uplifting way of dealing with the situation.

Charles Eisenstein points out how complicated and multi-layered the efforts to stabilize ecosystems, the climate situation, or similar challenges are, and how "simple," straightforward, and general—therefore also popular—the destruction or combating of specific "viruses" seems. He elaborates—as other authors have done before—on the dangerous transformation of society that this may initiate:

> I am sure that many of the control measures in force today will be partially relaxed in a few months. Partially relaxed, but ready-to-hand at any moment. As long as contagious diseases circulate, it is not unlikely that they will be enacted again and again in the future, or we will impose them on ourselves as new habits. As Deborah Tannen writes in a *Politico* article about the ongoing changes the coronavirus will bring to the world, "We now know that touching things, being around other people, and breathing air indoors can be risky.... It could become second nature to shy away from shaking hands or touching faces, and the way we wash our hands nonstop, you might fear we're all falling prey to a collective obsessive-compulsive disorder." After millennia, indeed millions of years of touch, contact, and togetherness,

does humanity's progress culminate in ceasing such activities because they are too risky?

The perspectives voiced by Eisenstein and other critical authors, which are anything but "conspiracy theories," must, in my opinion, become familiar in "Free Waldorf Schools" as a part of a progressive civil society of the near future—as must the whole problem of modern biotechnology in connection with the possibilities of digital control and surveillance. "What is at stake," the pedagogue Bernd Ruf recently wrote, is the "one-sidedness of a materialistic-reductionist, scientific-technical understanding of the human being and the world, and the attempt at its brute implementation in social norms."

I would like to emphasize that it is by no means necessary for the teaching staff to be experts in all these areas of concern; however, they, or parents, can and should invite knowledgeable speakers and be aware of the fact that they also have a clear *educational mission* with regard to the current, existential crisis. In this context, I do not view this educational mission and this educational opportunity as belonging exclusively within the school curriculum. Rather, I would like to remind you that one hundred years ago in the Stuttgart Waldorf School, "Free University Courses" were sometimes held in the evenings, with highly interesting speakers and topics, including loaded questions of contemporary history. Attendance at these events for students was of course voluntary, but the upper school students and parents were also invited—and of course the teachers (many of whom themselves also lectured and held discussions during these evenings). I think this is a model for the future; the broadening of horizons and intellectual discourse certainly benefits the school; we have the necessary spaces and opportunities—and the students thus see us wrestling with present and future questions, educating ourselves further without being omniscient. Some of the students would certainly join us and the school would become more interesting and open—not just "school" in the traditional sense.

Insofar as Waldorf schools—in the sense of their founding principles—really see themselves as innovative, future-oriented, and socially conscious places for individual maturity and personal development, as institutions in which the "courage to tell the truth" is the first priority—also pedagogically—then in my opinion, they cannot avoid a differentiated contextual analysis of the complex "Covid" phenomenon; they owe this analysis of the situation not least to the children and young people to whom they want and have to impart an orientation—an *orientation to reality*, which is of fundamental importance for the adolescent's developing *trust* in life and in the world (Constanza Kaliks). I think that the necessary analysis of the situation is a positive and constructive responsibility, in the sense mentioned above, a responsibility that does not increase the already existing demand to an inordinate degree but rather leads deeper into the subject matter and creates social objectivity and perspective.

By raising the level of knowledge and thoughtful reflection beyond the sphere of the daily news, not only can the divisions within school communities and the tendency toward silencing certain viewpoints be overcome, but also highly interesting and future-oriented lessons will emerge. If, for example, one deals with the ecological background of serious infectious diseases—I refer to the excellent contributions of the physicians Matthias Girke and Georg Soldner, as well as the farmers and environmentalists Ueli Hurter and Jean-Michel Florin in their new Goetheanum book on the Covid challenge—one becomes very awake to the complex difficulty of the situation that humanity is facing and that it has to solve, and by no means only in a superficial way (through maximum protection from viruses). If one delves into these contexts, one comes to a better understanding of the situation and gradually regains one's own power of judgment—indeed, one's own thinking, which in recent months has seemed to be switched off in many people, spellbound by media reports and knee-jerk responses, panic and absolute compliance or denial.

As I said, there is an undoubted opportunity for orientation in real discussion and deepening, and we could, with the Waldorf school communities, take on a social model function of paradigm-spanning, multi-perspective education, which is lacking everywhere. In fact, we must attempt to qualitatively grasp the "spiritual character of the overall situation" at a much higher level.

Second, I am of the opinion that it has been one of the tasks of the Waldorf School since its founding in the fall of 1919 to advocate vigorously, both within and outside the school walls, for the threatened qualities of childhood and youth development. Rudolf Steiner explained internally, but also publicly with impressive research results, the importance of imitation and trust, face-to-face encounter, composure, closeness and community, movement, music, creativity, and religion for the healthy development of the child. He also worked out which immediate relationship qualities play a decisive role in this, how resilience and salutogenesis, the acquisition of mental and bodily health—instead of pathologization and traumatization—can be assessed, and the first Waldorf teachers in turn also spoke openly on these themes in publications and at conferences.

From the beginning, the protection of childhood was one of the essential goals of the Waldorf School. "We must give the children back their childhood!" said Rudolf Steiner; this also meant the protection of children from state, economic, industrial, and other interests. From the beginning, it was one of the basic concerns of Waldorf schools to promote the social and ecological co-responsibility of children and adolescents and not the fear of the other, to promote connection with the world instead of withdrawal and "safe" isolation—and these perspectives were also publicly advocated by Steiner and the college of teachers. This is also needed today and in a decisive way, more than ever before. It must become very clear in the future that parents and teachers are not willing to surrender the essentials of childhood and child development—and that they demand society-wide solutions to ecological and medical problems, rather than merely treating the symptoms with "protective" measures such as distancing and isolation.

Third, I am convinced that the school communities of the "Free Waldorf Schools" must become much more real in the future. In accordance with its conception, the Waldorf school community should develop on a small scale a model for the responsible civil society of the future, in which each individual participates in a co-creative way, especially on essential questions. "We need transparent and public debate for all the issues at hand, the weighing of different paths, and, in the end, the greatest possible participation of people themselves in making decisions. This will not come by itself. Rather, we have to fight for it," writes Gerald Häfner with regard to the civic challenges of the present and near future. This also applies to Waldorf school communities.

As in the present crisis, spontaneous associations can form of individual, committed parents and teachers, which are not organized in the sense of the representative system but which are binding and at the same time proceed in an extraordinarily flexible, problem-oriented and active way, seeking creative solutions or at least improvisations in a difficult time—dissolving the classical dichotomy of teacher and parent roles (and "representatives" standing in between). Jan Göschen, drawing on new sociopsychological literature, recently described how "disaster communities" or "grassroots" initiatives can form in a self-organized manner in times of crisis, with a great degree of mutual support among those involved, and how they create and seize free spaces, react quickly, and are capable of action. However, he also described what happens when superordinate governing bodies experience such initiatives only as a disturbance and a threat to their central planning and control, which they in turn exercise in the sense of state-directed specifications within the school, in a "top-down" manner (according to the model of "command and control").

The already unstable school community can finally break apart as a result of such a split; however, the entire problem that becomes manifest can also be used as an occasion to pose the question of communal organization in a completely new way and, as in society as a whole, "create new forms of participation and decision-making" (Häfner). In this lies a great, essential opportunity for the future. School communities do exist at Waldorf schools—in contrast to the situation at many state-run *Gymnasien*, *Realschulen*, or *Hauptschulen*.* Developing and expanding them is of great importance.

---

* In Germany, *Hauptschule* is the vocational path, *Realschule* is geared toward the more advanced technical trades, and *Gymnasium* is the preparatory path for university.

Fourth, in my opinion, the current crisis offers the possibility—but also makes it necessary—to once again raise the question of the spiritual core and inner identity, as well as the social and spiritual identity, of Waldorf schools. This means, at the same time: to raise the question of the meaning of Anthroposophy and the anthroposophic study of the human being for the colleges of teachers and schools that exist today. If the existential threat to Waldorf schools that has now emerged cannot be mastered by waiting and standing still, by silence and adaptation—for which there is much to be said—then it is necessary to actively engage, in full consciousness, with the debate over the significance and value of Anthroposophy.

I hope to have shown in one of my recent books that this holds true also with regard to the accusation of racism and anti-Semitism against Rudolf Steiner and Anthroposophy.* We are not preparing for the future if we more or less silently accept and sidestep insinuations and accusations of this kind, or avoid this difficult topic (or even the overall topic of "Rudolf Steiner and Anthroposophy") in Waldorf schools, if we pretend to be "free" of it, if we ignore or court critics; nor are we preparing for the future by so rarely addressing the spiritual foundations of Waldorf education—which are *diametrically* opposed to racist, anti-Semitic, inhuman, and totalitarian thinking—and with such

---

* See Peter Selg, *Anthroposophy and the Accusation of Racism: Society and Medicine in a Totalitarian Age*, trans. J. Martin (Hudson, NY: SteinerBooks, 2022).

restraint, as has been done recently in many schools with regard to the public, but also with regard to the school's own "public" of parents and students. The Berlin teacher Ernst Weissert spoke in retrospect of a "significant concentration on the core of the school," a new "reflection on Rudolf Steiner's study of the human being," and the "methods of the new art of education" in the difficult time of National Socialism—a reflection on the "spiritual core" of the Waldorf School. What was demonstrably successful at that time—even if only in the secrecy of small communities or at least in the consciousness of many involved—should today, under much more favorable circumstances, without prohibition and persecution, by no means be overlooked—and it indeed seems to me to be an existential need, in the true sense of the words, and instrumental in forming identity and continuity.

One can describe such a necessity, I think, with the simple term "civil courage." This is commonly understood to mean the courage of people to make their own judgments and to stand up for social values, for human dignity, human rights, and democracy—without regard for possible reactions from the public or the authorities. Waldorf teachers, as I hope has become clear through the first part of my presentation, had certainly developed such an understanding of "civil courage" from 1933 to 1941 in their school buildings, in the *inner space of their pedagogy*, within their teaching and education, which they uncompromisingly continued in the spirit of their anthroposophic and humanistic values, although they did not have a completely homogeneous parent body and therefore took a not inconsiderable risk (as the fate of Hans Rutz, among others, shows). Nowadays, in the Covid situation and in our democratic state system, the schools must, in my opinion, also *publicly* develop such civil courage, although this can make them the target of many defamatory attacks that have been flying around the ears of Anthroposophy and anthroposophic institutions for decades—from alleged "occultism" to supposed collaboration with right-wing extremist forces. In the midst of a digitalized world, we must stand up anew with all vigor and with all civil courage for the essence and dignity of the human being, our relationships and encounters, our trust in life and the world— and we *can* do this. The children and the "pedagogical spaces"—the real ones, not the virtual ones—need our protection, our defense, and our courage, in the "sense of responsibility for the whole."

Certainly, Waldorf schools are also subject to legal regulations and official orders. But the deeper and the more subtly these intervene in the core areas of pedagogical responsibility and child development, the more do concrete organizational tasks arise for Waldorf schools. Educators and parents cannot step out of this difficult responsibility by merely making room for state action. Such inaction would not be neutral but fatal; it would be the opposite of what children need and what Waldorf education is all about. "What comes out of a crisis is up to us. The way we understand a crisis as well as the resolutions we make in the face of it, help to determine it," writes Gerald Häfner. "*We must indeed give children back their childhood! That is a task of the Waldorf School*" (Rudolf Steiner).

Bibliography

Deuchert, Norbert. "Zur Geschichte der Waldorfschule 1933–1940" [On the history of the Waldorf School] and "Der Kampf um die Waldorfschule im Nationalsozialismus" [The struggle for the Waldorf School under National Socialism].In *Berichtsheft des Bundes der Freien Waldorfschulen* [Reports of the Federation of Independent Waldorf Schools] (Stuttgart: Dec. 1984/87). Reprinted in *Flensburger Hefte*, no. 8, (1991), pp. 95–130.

Eisenstein, Charles, Thomas Hardtmuth, Christoph Hueck, and Andreas Neider. *Corona und die Überwindung der Getrenntheit: Neue medizinische, politische, kulturelle und anthroposophische Aspekte der Corona-Pandemie* [Covid and the overcoming of separateness: New medical, political, cultural, and anthroposophical aspects of the Covid pandemic] (Stuttgart: Akanthos Akademie für anthroposophische Forschung und Entwicklung, 2020).

Florin, Jean-Michel. "Corona and Biodynamic Agriculture," in *Perspectives and Initiatives in the Times of Coronavirus*. Ed. Ueli Hurter and Justus Wittich, trans. C. Howard (Forest Row, UK: Rudolf Steiner Press, 2020).

Frielingsdorf, Volker. *Geschichte der Waldorfpädagogik: Von ihrem Ursprung bis zur Gegenwart* [History of Waldorf education: From its origins to the present] (Weinheim: Beltz GmbH, 2019), chap. 3, "Bedrohung, Existenzgefährdung und Schließung der Waldorfschulen im Dritten Reich (1933–1945)" [Endangerment, existential threat, and closure of Waldorf schools in the Third Reich (1933–1945)], pp. 153–202.

Girke, Matthias and Georg Soldner. "Consequences of Covid-19 – Perspectives of Anthroposophic Medicine," in *Perspectives and Initiatives in the Times of Coronavirus*. Ed. U. Hurter and J. Wittich (Forest Row, UK: Rudolf Steiner Press, 2020).

Göschel, Jan. "Consequences of Covid 19 – The Perspective of
Anthroposophic Curative Education, Social Pedagogy,
Social Therapy, and Inclusive Social Development." In
Perspectives and Initiatives in the Times of Corona. Ed.
U. Hurter and J. Wittich, trans. C. Howard (Forest Row,
UK: Rudolf Steiner Press, 2020).

Götte, Wenzel M. *Erfahrungen mit Schulautonomie: Das
Beispiel der Freien Waldorfschulen* [Experiences with
school autonomy: The example of the independent Waldorf
schools]. PhD diss., University of Bielefeld, June 2000
(Stuttgart: Freies Geistesleben, 2006).

Häfner, Gerald. "Understanding History from the Future – Crisis
as Opportunity." In *Perspectives and Initiatives in the
Times of Corona*. Ed. U. Hurter and J. Wittich, trans.
C. Howard (Forest Row, UK: Rudolf Steiner Press, 2020).

Haid, Christiane. "The Hidden Sun – Reality, Language, and
Art in Corona Times." In *Perspectives and Initiatives in
the Times of Corona*. Ed. U. Hurter and J. Wittich, trans.
C. Howard (Forest Row, UK: Rudolf Steiner Press, 2020).

Hurter, Ueli and Jean-Michel Florin. "Challenges and
Perspectives of the Corona Crisis in the Agricultural and
Food Industry." In *Perspectives and Initiatives in the Times
of Corona*. Ed. U. Hurter and J. Wittich, trans. C. Howard
(Forest Row, UK: Rudolf Steiner Press, 2020).

Husemann, Armin. *Seelische Störungen bei Erwachsenen
nach in der Kindheit erlittener nationalsozialistischer
Verfolgung* [Mental disorders in adults following Nazi
persecution suffered in childhood], PhD diss., University
of Tübingen, 1980.

———. "Medical Thinking and Medical Practice," in *Form, Life,
and Consciousness: An Introduction to Anthroposophic
Medicine* (Hudson, NY: Steiner Books, 2019).

Kaliks, Constanza. "Aspects of Dealing with the Corona Crisis
for Youth," in *Perspectives and Initiatives in the Times of
Corona*. Ed. U. Hurter and J. Wittich, trans. Youth Section
members (Forest Row, UK: Rudolf Steiner Press, 2020).

Lobo, Sascha. *Realitätsschock: Zehn Lehren aus der Gegenwart* [Reality shock: Ten lessons from the present] (Cologne: Kiepenheuer und Witsch GmbH, 2019).

Priestman, Karen. *Illusion of Coexistence: The Waldorf Schools in the Third Reich, 1933–1941*. PhD diss., Wilfried Laurier University, 2009.

Röh, Claus-Peter and Florian Osswald. "Education in Times of Corona." In *Perspectives and Initiatives in the Times of Corona*. Ed. U. Hurter and J. Wittich, trans. C. Howard (Forest Row: Rudolf Steiner Press, 2020).

Ruf, Bernd. "'Denn wenn ihr nicht Nein sagt.…' Von der Kindheit in der Coronakrise und dem Mut des Lehrers zur Wahrheit" ["'For if you do not say no.…' On childhood in the Corona crisis and the teachers' courage for the truth"]. In *Das Goetheanum: Wochenschrift für Anthroposophie*, no. 22, May 29, 2020, pp. 6–9.

——. *Educating Traumatized Children: Waldorf Education in Crisis Intervention*. Great Barrington, MA: Lindisfarne Books, 2013.

Selg, Peter. *Anthroposophie und Waldorfpädagogik* [Anthroposophy and Waldorf education] (Arlesheim: Ita Wegman Institute, 2019).

——. *Erzwungene Schließung: Die Ansprachen der Stuttgarter Lehrer nach dem Ende der Waldorfschule im deutschen Faschismus (1938)* [Forced closure: The speeches of the Stuttgart teachers after the end of the Waldorf school under German fascism (1938)] (Arlesheim: Ita Wegman Institute, 2019).

——. *The Essence of Waldorf Education*. Trans. M. Saar (Great Barrington, MA: SteinerBooks, 2010).

——. *Die Intentionen Ita Wegmans: 1925–1943* [The intentions of Ita Wegman: 1925–1943] (Arlesheim: Ita Wegman Institute, 2019).

———. "A Medicalized Society?" In *The Mystery of the Earth: Essays in the Time of Coronavirus.* Trans. M. V. Miller and D. E. Miller (Hudson, NY: SteinerBooks, 2021).

———. *The Mystery of the Earth: Essays in the Time of Coronavirus.* Trans. M. V. Miller and D. E. Miller (Hudson, NY: SteinerBooks, 2021).

———. *After Auschwitz: Reflections on the Future of Medicine* (Hudson, NY: SteinerBooks, 2022).

———. *Anthroposophy and the Accusation of Racism: Society and Medicine in a Totalitarian Age* (Hudson, NY: SteinerBooks, 2022).

———. *Rudolf Steiner: Life and Work.* Trans. M. Saar, 7 vols. (Great Barrington, MA: SteinerBooks, 2014–19).

———. *Der Untergang des Abendlands? Rudolf Steiners Auseinandersetzung mit Oswald Spengler* [The decline of the West? Rudolf Steiner's engagement with Oswald Spengler] (Arlesheim and Dornach: Verlag am Goetheanum and Verlag des Ita Wegmans Institute, 2020).

Steiner, Rudolf. *Becoming the Archangel Michael's Companions: Rudolf Steiner's Challenge to the Younger Generation* CW 217 (Great Barrington, MA: SteinerBooks, 2007).

———. *Education for Adolesents* CW 302 (Hudson, NY: Anthroposophic Press, 1996).

———. *Mantric Sayings: Meditations 1903–1925* CW 268 (Great Barrington, MA: SteinerBooks, 2015).

———. *Michael's Mission: Revealing the Essential Secrets of Human Nature* CW 194 (Forest Row, UK: Rudolf Steiner Press, 2016).

———. *Neugestaltung des sozialen Organismus* [The new formation of the social organism] CW 330 (Basel: Rudolf Steiner Verlag, 1983).

———. *On Epidemics: Spiritual Perspectives* (selections from the work of Rudolf Steiner) (Forest Row, UK: Rudolf Steiner Press, 2012).

———. *Problems of Society: An Esoteric View: From Luciferic Past to Ahrimanic Future* CW 193 (Forest Row, UK: Rudolf Steiner Press, 2016).

———. *The Renewal of the Social Organism* CW 24 (Spring Valley, NY: Anthroposophic Press, 1985).

———. *Supersensible Knowledge* CW 55 (Hudson, NY: Anthroposophic Press, 1987).

Wember, Valentin. *Was will Waldorf wirklich? Die unbekannte Erziehungskunst Rudolf Steiners* [What does Waldorf really want? The unknown art of education of Rudolf Steiner] (Tübingen: Stratos Verlag, 2019).

Werner, Uwe. *Anthroposophen in der Zeit des Nationalsozialismus (1933—1945)* [Anthroposophists in the time of National Socialism (1933–1945)] (Munich: Oldenbourg Wissenschaftsverlag, 1999), pp. 94–139, 207–241.

———. *Waldorfschulen im nationalsozialistischen Deutschland: Eine kleine Monografie* [Waldorf schools in National Socialist Germany: A small monograph] (Hamburg: Pädagogische Forschungsstelle Stuttgart, 2017).

Zweig, Stefan. *The World of Yesterday: An Autobiography* (Lincoln, NE: University of Nebraska, 1964).

Endnotes

1   See Addendum.

2   See Peter Selg, *The Mystery of the Earth: Essays in the Time of Coronavirus*, trans. M. V. Miller and D. E. Miller (Hudson, NY: SteinerBooks, 2021).

3   See Hurter, Ueli, and Jean-Michel Florin, *Perspectives and Initiatives in the Times of Corona*, ed. U. Hurter and J. Wittich, trans. C. Howard (Forest Row, UK: Rudolf Steiner Press, 2020).

4   See Peter Selg, *Ein Brückenschlag zum Rechtsextremismus? Über die Anthroposophie in der Zeit des Nationalsozialismus* [A bridge to right-wing extremism? On Anthroposophy in the time of National Socialism] (Arlesheim, CH: Ita Wegman Institute, 2021).

5   Rudolf Steiner, lecture of June 17, 1921, in *Education for Adolesents* (CW 302), trans. C. Hoffman (Hudson, NY: Anthroposophic Press, 1996).

6   Rudolf Steiner, June 1, 1919, *Education as a Force for Social Change* (CW 296), trans. R. F. Lathe and N. P. Whittaker (Hudson, NY: Anthroposophic Press, 1997).

7   See Addendum.

8   Amartya Sen, "Die Pandemie des Autoritarismus" [The pandemic of authoritarianism], in *Blätter für deutsche und internationale Politik* (Dec. 2020), p. 100.

9   Ita Wegman to Ernst Lehrs, Jan. 20, 1931. Ita Wegman Archive, Arlesheim; in Peter Selg, *A Grand Metamorphosis: Contributions to a Spiritual-Scientific Anthropology and Education of Adolescents*, trans. M. Saar (Great Barrington, MA: SteinerBooks, 2008).

10 Georg Soldner, "Ökologie und Pandemie: Was lernen wir an Covid-19?" [Ecology and pandemic: What can we learn from Covid-19?], https://medsektion-goetheanum.org/.

11   Charles Eisenstein, "Extinction and the Revolution of Love" (Jan. 2020), https://charleseisenstein.org/essays/extinction-and-the-revolution-of-love/.

12   Navid Kermani, "Der fremde Blick" ["The Foreign View"], in *Frankfurter Allgemeine Zeitung*, Nov. 7, 2020.

13   Soldner, "Ökologie."

14   PWC and UBS, "Riding the Storm: Market turbulence accelerates diverging fortunes" (Oct. 2020); https://www.pwc.ch/en/insights/fs/billionaires-insights-2020.html.

15   Thomas Hardtmuth, *Das Corona-Syndrom—warum die Angst gefährlicher ist als das Virus* [The Covid syndrome—Why fear is more dangerous than the virus], in Charles Eisenstein, et al., *Corona und die Überwindung der Getrenntheit: Neue medizinische, politische, kulturelle und anthroposophische Aspekte der Corona-Pandemie* [Covid and the overcoming of separateness: New medical, political, cultural, and anthroposophical aspects of the Covid pandemic] (Stuttgart: Akanthos Akademie für anthroposophische Forschung und Entwicklung, 2020).

16   Kermani, "Der Fremde Blick."

17   Soldner, "Ökologie."

18   Paul Schreyer, *Chronik einer angekündigten Krise: Wie ein Virus die Welt verändern konnte* [Chronicle of an announced crisis: How a virus was able to change the world] (Berlin: Westend Verlag GmbH, 2020).

19   Ibid., p. 51.

20   Ibid., p. 40.

21   Ibid., p. 45.

22   Ibid., p. 35.

23   Richard A. Clarke, "Finding the Right Balance against Bioterrorism," *Emerging Infectious Diseases*, vol. 5, no. 4 (Aug. 1999), p. 497.

24   Schreyer, *Chronik*, p. 46.

25 Ibid., p. 58.

26 Ibid., p. 58f.

27 Ibid., p. 60.

28 Ibid., p. 61.

29 Ibid., p. 63.

30 Rockefeller Foundation, "Scenarios for the Future of Technology and International Development" (May 2010), p. 18ff.

31 Schreyer, *Chronik*, p. 87.

32 Ibid., p. 98.

33 Ibid., p. 99.

34 Event 201, Event 201 Recommendations, "Public-private Cooperation for Pandemic Preparedness and Response – A Call to Action," https://www.centerforhealthsecurity.org /event201/recommendations.html.

35 Norbert Häring, "Lock Step – The eerily prescient pandemic scenario of the Rockefeller Foundation," *Money and More* (May 12, 2020), https://norberthaering.de/en /power-control/lock-step-rockefeller/.

36 Schreyer, *Chronik*, p. 160.

37 Ibid.

38 Ibid., p. 71.

39 Clemens G. Arvay, *Wir können es besser: Wie Umweltzerstörung die Corona-Pandemie auslöste und warum ökologische Medizin unsere Rettung ist* [We can do better: How environmental destruction triggered the Covid pandemic and why ecological medicine is our salvation] (Cologne: Quadriga, 2020).

40 Ibid., p. 143.

41 Ibid., p. 22.

42 Hardtmuth, *Das Corona-Syndrom*, p. 39. See note 15.

43   Sen, "Die Pandemie des Autoritarismus," p. 100; see note 8.

44   See note 11.

45   Stefan Zweig, *Worte haben keine Macht mehr: Essays zu Politik und Zeitgeschehen* [Words no longer have power: Essays on politics and contemporary events] (Vienna: Sonderzahl, 2019), p. 59.

46   See *Warum schweigen die Lämmer? Wie Elitendemokratie und Neoliberalismus unsere Gesellschaft und unsere Lebensgrundlagen zerstören* [Why are the lambs silent? How elite democracy and neoliberalism destroy our society and our livelihoods] (Frankfurt: Westend Westend Verlag GmbH, 2019).

47   Schreyer, *Chronik*, p. 21.

48   Charles Eisenstein, "Extinction and the Revolution of Love," January 2020, https://charleseisenstein.org/essays/extinction-and-the-revolution-of-love/.

49   Thomas Fuchs, *In Defense of the Human Being: Foundational Questions of an Embodied Anthropology*, (New York and London: Oxford University, 2021), p. 23.

50   Ibid., p. 44.

51   Jochen Krautz, "Bildendes Lernen braucht Schule und Unterricht" [Educational learning requires school and teaching], in *Lockdown 2020: Wie ein Virus dazu benutzt wird, die Gesellschaft zu verändern* [Lockdown 2020: How a virus is being used to change society], eds. Hannes Hofbauer and Stefan Kraft (Vienna: Promedia, 2020), p. 226f.

52   Ibid., p. 223.

53   Fuchs, *In Defense of the Human Being*, p. 1.

54   Hannes Hofbauer and Stefan Kraft, ed. *Lockdown 2020: Wie ein Virus dazu benutzt wird, die Gesellschaft zu verändern* [Lockdown 2020: How a virus is being used to change society] (Vienna: Promedia, 2020), pp. 11–127; see also Peter Selg, "A Medicalized Society?" in *The Mystery*

of the Earth: Essays in the Time of Coronavirus, trans. M. Miller and D. Miller (Hudson, NY: SteinerBooks, 2021).

55   Sascha Lobo, *Realitätsschock: Zehn Lehren aus der Gegenwart* [Reality shock: Ten lessons from the present] (Cologne: Kiepenheuer und Witsch GmbH, 2019), p. 197.

56   Ibid., p. 201.

57   Ibid., p. 203.

58   Ibid., p. 208.

59   Ibid., p. 209.

60   Ibid., p. 211.

61   Fuchs, *In Defense of the Human Being*, p. 3.

62   Yuval Noah Harari, *Homo Deus: A Brief History of Tomorrow* (New York: HarperCollins, 2017).

63   Ibid.

64   Fuchs, *In Defense of the Human Being*, p. 58.

65   Werner Pluta, "Elon Musk will Mensch und KI Vereinen," Golem.de, July 17, 2019, https://www.golem.de/news /neuralink-elon-musk-will-mensch-und-ki-vereinen-1907 -142614.html.

66   Fuchs, *In Defense of the Human Being*, p. 8.

67   Klaus Schwab and Thierry Malleret, *Covid-19: The Great Reset* (Geneva, CH: World Economic Forum, 2020). See, e.g., Peter Selg, *The Future of Ahriman and the Awakening of Souls: The Spirit-Presence of the Mystery Dramas*, trans. P. King (Forest Row, UK: Temple Lodge Publications, 2022).

68   Rudolf Steiner, May 22, 1919, in *Betriebsräte und Sozialisierung. Diskussionsabende mit den Arbeiterausschüssen der großen Betriebe Stuttgarts, 1919* [Works councils and socialization: Discussion evenings with the workers' committees of Stuttgart's large factories, 1919] (CW 331), not available in English. See also Peter Selg, "Rudolf Steiners Einsatz für die Gegenwart und Zukunft

der sozialen Dreigliederung" [Rudolf Steiner's commitment
to the present and future of social threefolding], in Peter
Selg and Marc Desaules, *Ökonomie der Brüderlichkeit:
Zur Aktualität der sozialen Dreigliederung* [Economy
of fraternity: On the topicality of social threefolding]
(Arlesheim: Ita Wegman Institute, 2017).

69   Schreyer, *Chronik*, p. 16. See note 18.

70   Hardtmuth, *Das Corona-Syndrom*, p. 44; see note 15.

71   Schreyer, *Chronik*, p. 155.

72   Sascha Lobo, *Realitätsschock*, p. 220.

73   Amartya Sen, "Die Pandemie des Autoritarismus," p. 100.
     See note 8.

74   Martin Buber, "Elements of the Interhuman," in *The
     Knowledge of Man: Selected Essays*, ed. M. Friedman,
     trans. M. Friedman and R. G. Smith (New York: Harper
     and Row, 1965), pp. 78–79.

75   Ibid., p. 79.

76   Stephan Lessenich, *Grenzen der Demokrati: Teilhabe als
     Verteilungsproblem* [Limits of democracy: Participation as
     a problem of distribution] (Stuttgart: Reclam Verlag, 2019),
     p. 33.

77   Ivan Illich, *Medical Nemesis: The Expropriation of Health*
     (New York: Random House, 1976), p. 7.

78   Fuchs, *In Defense of the Human Being*, p. 6. See note 49.

79   Christoph Hueck, *Impfung, Impfnachweis, Impfpflicht—
     Ideologie der Kontrolle versus christlicher Individualismus*
     [Vaccination, proof of vaccination, compulsory
     vaccination—Ideology of control versus Christian
     individualism], in Charles Eisenstein, et al., *Corona und
     die Überwindung der Getrenntheit: Neue medizinische,
     politische, kulturelle und anthroposophische Aspekte
     der Corona-Pandemie* [Corona and the Overcoming
     of Separateness: New medical, political, cultural, and
     anthroposophical aspects of the Corona pandemic]

(Stuttgart: Akanthos Akademie für anthroposophische
Forschung und Entwicklung, 2020), p. 66.

80   Rudolf Steiner, *Mantric Sayings: Meditations 1903–1925*
(CW 268), trans. D. L. Fleming and C. Bamford (Great
Barrington, MA: SteinerBooks, 2015), p. 105.

81   Rudolf Steiner, Aug. 9, 1919, in *Education as a Social
Force for Change* (CW 296), trans. R. F. Lathe and N. P.
Whittaker (Hudson, NY: Anthroposophic Press, 1997).

82   Rudolf Steiner, Oct. 7, 1922, in *Becoming the Archangel
Michael's Companions: Rudolf Steiner's Challenge to
the Younger Generation* (CW 217), trans. R. M. Querido
(Great Barrington, MA: SteinerBooks, 2007), p. 55.

83   Rudolf Steiner, Feb. 28, 1907, in *Supersensible Knowledge*
(CW 55), trans. R. Stebbing (Hudson, NY: Anthroposophic
Press, 1987), p. 139.

84   Charles Eisenstein, "Extinction and the Revolution of
Love," Jan. 2020, https://charleseisenstein.org/essays
/extinction-and-the-revolution-of-love/.

85   Navid Kermani, "Der fremde Blick" [The foreign view], in
Frankfurter Allgemeine Zeitung, Nov. 7, 2020.

86   See Peter Selg, *Rudolf Steiner: Life and Work, Vol. 5,
1919–1922: Social Threefolding and the Waldorf School*,
trans. M. Saar (Great Barrington, MA: SteinerBooks,
2017).

87   See Peter Selg, *The Essence of Waldorf Education*, trans.
M. Saar (Great Barrington, MA: SteinerBooks, 2010).

88   Rudolf Steiner, lecture three (Aug. 31, 1919), in *The
Spirit of the Waldorf School*, trans. R. E. Lathe and N. P.
Whittaker (Hudson, NY: Anthroposophic Press, 1995).

89   Rudolf Steiner, *The Renewal of the Social Organism* (CW
24), trans. E. Bowen-Wedgewood and R. Mariott (Spring
Valley, NY: Anthroposophic Press, 1985).

90   Rudolf Steiner, lecture of Aug. 2, 1922, in *Rethinking
Economics: Lectures and Seminars on World Economics*

(CW 340/341), trans. A. O. Barfield and T. Gordon-Jones (Great Barrington, MA: SteinerBooks, 2013).

91   Rudolf Steiner, lecture of Dec. 12, 1918, in *Die soziale Grundforderung unserer Zeit – In geänderter Zeitlage* [The fundamental social demand of our time: In the changed conditions of the time] (GA 186). Part of this volume of The Collected Works of Rudolf Steiner is available in English as *The Challenge of the Times*.

92   Rudolf Steiner, Apr. 25, 1919, *Neugestaltung des sozialen Organismus* [The new formation of the social organism] (CW 330) (Rudolf Steiner Verlag, 1983), not in English.

93   Rudolf Steiner, lecture of Sept. 13, 1919, in *Problems of Society: And Esoteric View: From Luciferic Past to Ahrimanic Future* (CW 193), trans. M. Barton (Forest Row, UK: Rudolf Steiner Press, 2016).

94   Rudolf Steiner, lecture of Dec. 14, 1919, in *Michael's Mission: Revealing the Essential Secrets of Human Nature* (CW 194), trans. J. Collis (Forest Row, UK: Rudolf Steiner Press, 2016).

95   Charles Eisenstein, "The Coronation," (March 2020), https://charleseisenstein.org/essays/the-coronation/.

Books by Peter Selg
in English Translation

On Rudolf Steiner

Rudolf Steiner: Life and Work (1924–1925): The Anthroposophical Society and the School for Spiritual Science, vol. 7 of 7 (2019)

Spiritual Friendship: Rudolf Steiner and Christian Morgenstern (2018)

Rudolf Steiner: Life and Work (1923): The Burning of the Goetheanum, vol. 6 of 7 (2018)

Rudolf Steiner: Life and Work (1919–1922): Social Threefolding and the Waldorf School, vol. 5 of 7 (2017)

Rudolf Steiner: Life and Work (1914–1918): The Years of World War I , vol. 4 of 7 (2016)

Rudolf Steiner: Life and Work (1900–1914): Spiritual Science and Spiritual Community, vol. 3 of 7 (2015)

Rudolf Steiner: Life and Work (1890–1900): Weimar and Berlin, vol. 2 of 7 (2014)

Rudolf Steiner: Life and Work (1861–1890): Childhood, Youth, and Study Years, vol. 1 of 7 (2014)

Rudolf Steiner and Christian Rosenkreutz (2012)

Rudolf Steiner as a Spiritual Teacher: From Recollections of Those Who Knew Him (2010)

On Christology

The Origins of the Creed of The Christian Community: Its History and Significance Today (2019)

Rudolf Steiner and The Christian Community (2018)

The Sufferings of the Nathan Soul: Anthroposophic Christology on the Eve of World War I (2016)

The Lord's Prayer and Rudolf Steiner: A Study of His Insights into the Archetypal Prayer of Christianity (2014)

The Creative Power of Anthroposophical Christology: An Outline of Occult Science · The First Goetheanum · The Fifth Gospel · The Christmas Conference (with Sergei O. Prokofieff) (2012)

Christ and the Disciples: The Destiny of an Inner Community (2012)

The Figure of Christ: Rudolf Steiner and the Spiritual Intention behind the Goetheanum's Central Work of Art (2009)

Rudolf Steiner and the Fifth Gospel: Insights into a New Understanding of the Christ Mystery (2010)

Seeing Christ in Sickness and Healing (2005)

ON GENERAL ANTHROPOSOPHY

The Mysteries of the Future: A Study of the work of Sergei O. Prokofieff, (2021)

The Anthroposophical Society: The Understanding and Continued Activity of the Christmas Conference, edited with Marc Desaules (2018)

The Warmth Meditation: A Path to the Good in the Service of Healing (2016)

The Michael School: And the School of Spiritual Science (2016)

The Destiny of the Michael Community: Foundation Stone for the Future (2014)

Spiritual Resistance: Ita Wegman 1933–1935 (2014)

The Last Three Years: Ita Wegman in Ascona, 1940–1943 (2014)

From Gurs to Auschwitz: The Inner Journey of Maria Krehbiel-Darmstädter (2013)

Crisis in the Anthroposophical Society: And Pathways to the Future, with Sergei O. Prokofieff (2013)

Rudolf Steiner's Foundation Stone Meditation: And the Destruction of the Twentieth Century (2013)

The Culture of Selflessness: Rudolf Steiner, the Fifth Gospel, and the Time of Extremes (2012)

The Mystery of the Heart: The Sacramental Physiology of the Heart in Aristotle, Thomas Aquinas, and Rudolf Steiner (2012)

Rudolf Steiner and the School for Spiritual Science: The Foundation of the "First Class" (2012)

Rudolf Steiner's Intentions for the Anthroposophical Society: The Executive Council, the School for Spiritual Science, and the Sections (2011)

The Fundamental Social Law: Rudolf Steiner on the Work of the Individual and the Spirit of Community (2011)

The Path of the Soul after Death: The Community of the Living and the Dead as Witnessed by Rudolf Steiner in his Eulogies and Farewell Addresses (2011)

The Agriculture Course, Koberwitz, Whitsun 1924: Rudolf Steiner and the Beginnings of Biodynamics (2010)

ON ANTHROPOSOPHICAL MEDICINE
AND CURATIVE EDUCATION

Anthroposophy and the Accusation of Racism: Society and Medicine in a Totalitarian Age (2022)

After Auschwitz: Reflections on the Future of Medicine (2022)

The Mystery of the Earth: Essays in the Time of Coronavirus (2021)

Honoring Life: Medical Ethics and Physician-Assisted Suicide, with Sergei O. Prokofieff (2014)

I Am for Going Ahead: Ita Wegman's Work for the Social Ideals of Anthroposophy (2012)

The Child with Special Needs: Letters and Essays on Curative Education (ed.) (2009)

Ita Wegman and Karl König: Letters and Documents (2008)

Karl König's Path to Anthroposophy (2008)

Karl König: My Task: Autobiography and Biographies (ed.) (2008)

ON CHILD DEVELOPMENT
AND WALDORF EDUCATION

The Child as a Sense Organ: An Anthroposophic Understanding of Imitation Processes (2017)

I Am Different from You: How Children Experience Themselves and the World in the Middle of Childhood (2011)

Unbornness: Human Preexistence and the Journey toward Birth (2010)

The Essence of Waldorf Education (2010)

The Therapeutic Eye: How Rudolf Steiner Observed Children (2008)

A Grand Metamorphosis: Contributions to the Spiritual–scientific Anthropology and Education of Adolescents (2008)

RECENT BOOKS BY THIS AUTHOR

Anthroposophy and the Accusation of Racism
Society and Medicine in a Totalitarian Age

Peter Selg

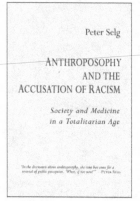

The original subtitle of Rudolf Stein-er's *Philosophy of Freedom* ("the basis for a modern worldview") points to the lifelong project with which he was engaged—lay-ing the foundation so that people today can comprehend the world in which we live, beginning with our-selves as individual, utterly unique embodiments of humanity.

It's a spiritual worldview born of the essence of the modern scientific reckoning with knowledge. But its detrac-tors, critics, and outright opponents, speaking from the standpoint of other worldviews and denying the validity of this one, from the early 1900s to today, have continued to portray it in a very different light. One such critic, typical of others, writing in 2019, deemed it "dogmatic, irrational, anti-Enlightenment, racist."

With this book, Peter Selg addresses these and related issues head on.

ISBN 9781621482727 | pbk | 240 pgs

After Auschwitz

Reflections on the Future of Medicine

Peter Selg

Since 2009, Peter Selg, along with Polish historians, has led seminars on medical ethics at the Auschwitz-Birkenau memorial for students at Witten/Herdecke University, Germany. This book was created following a public event in 2019 that investigated the "lessons of Auschwitz" for the practice of medicine in society today and in the future.

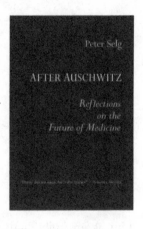

As well as commemorating the individual victims, the Auschwitz event focused on the role of German physicians in the Nazi regime. In this book, Dr. Selg's discussions go far beyond the historical events of the 1930s and '40s. Countering the legacy of Auschwitz-Birkenau and the inhumane medical practices of that time, he presents us with ways to advance forms of medicine today that encourage the most compassionate treatment of one another as human beings.

ISBN 9781621482666 | pbk | 282 pgs

Spiritual Friendship

Rudolf Steiner and Christian Morgenstern

Peter Selg

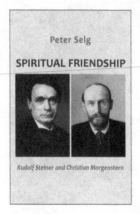

Peter Selg wrote this remarkable book on the formation of spiritual community and mutual assistance to coincide with the hundredth anniversary of Christian Morgenstern's death on March 31, 1914. Rudolf Steiner was, for Christian Morgenstern, the decisive spiritual teacher and facilitator of the future, both historically and to him as an individual, which is why Morgenstern wished to recommend Steiner for the Nobel Peace Prize. Rudolf Steiner felt great warmth of heart and gratitude toward Christian Morgenstern, his poetic work, and especially his groundbreaking way of working with anthroposophical Spiritual Science.

> "It is often said that to understand the poet we must go to his home country and understand that Christian Morgenstern is a poet of the spirit. And to understand this poet of the spirit, we must go into the land of spirit, to spirit regions."
>
> —Rudolf Steiner

ISBN 9781621482222 | pbk | 144 pgs

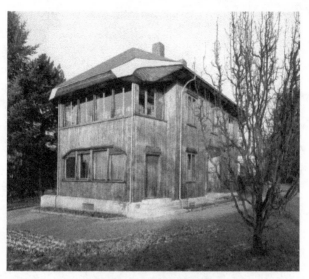

Ita Wegman Institute
for Basic Research into Anthroposophy

Pfeffinger Weg 1a, ch 4144 Arlesheim, Switzerland
www.wegmaninstitut.ch
e-mail: sekretariat@wegmaninstitut.ch

The Ita Wegman Institute for Basic Research into Anthroposophy is a not-for-profit research and teaching organization. It undertakes basic research into the lifework of Dr. Rudolf Steiner (1861–1925) and the application of Anthroposophy in specific areas of life, especially medicine, education, and curative education. Work carried out by the Institute is supported by a number of foundations and organizations and an international group of friends and supporters. The Director of the Institute is Prof. Dr. Peter Selg.